MANAGING QUALITY: STRATEGIC ISSUES IN HEALTH CARE MANAGEMENT

Managing Quality: Strategic Issues in Health Care Management

Edited by
HUW T.O. DAVIES, MANOUCHE TAVAKOLI,
MO MALEK and AILEEN R. NEILSON
*Department of Management, University of St Andrews,
Scotland*

Ashgate

Aldershot • Brookfield USA • Singapore • Sydney

Published by
Ashgate Publishing Limited
Gower House
Croft Road
Aldershot
Hampshire GU11 3HR
England

Ashgate Publishing Company
Old Post Road
Brookfield
Vermont 05036
USA

Ashgate website: http://www.ashgate.com

British Library Cataloguing in Publication Data
Managing quality : strategic issues in health care
    management
    1.Health services administration - Congresses 2.Total
    quality management in human services - Congresses
    I.Davies, Huw T. O.
    362.1'068

Library of Congress Catalog Card Number: 99-72982

ISBN 0 7546 1004 7

Printed and bound in Great Britain by MPG Books Ltd, Bodmin, Cornwall

Contents

List of Figures

List of Tables

Acknowledgments

We wish to thank, first of all, participants in the Third International Conference on *Strategic Issues in Health Care Management* held at the University of St Andrews, Scotland in April 1998. Despite inclement weather, their unfailing good humour and intellectual engagement ensured a productive and enjoyable time for all. We are particularly grateful to the session chairs, manuscript reviewers and contributors for their efforts in shaping the material in this volume.

Appreciation is also due to our colleagues in the PharmacoEconomics Research Centre, Department of Management, and School of Social Sciences, at the University of St Andrews. We are likewise grateful for the excellent support provided by Reprographics, Printing, and Residential and Business Services at St Andrews. These capable and friendly people assisted in preparing conference materials and ensured the smooth running of the conference. Mehran Zabihollah, Elizabeth Brock, Andrew Falconer and Fiona Spencer-Nairn also contributed to the conference management, and we thank them for their assistance.

Ann Hargreaves, Gail Gillespie and Elizabeth Brodie deserve a special mention for their assistance with all the organizational aspects of the conference and the production of this text. Unsung but not unappreciated.

Pat FitzGerald, Anne Keirby and Kate Trew contributed great skill and considerable patience in the preparation and publication of the text, and we thank them.

Regrettably, none of the above can be held responsible for the final product: this lies solely with the editors and the contributing authors.

Finally, Huw Davies would like to express his sincere gratitude to The Commonwealth Fund of New York City who funded a sabbatical in the United States. This manuscript was finalized during that period.

Huw T.O. Davies
Manouche Tavakoli
Mo Malek
Aileen R. Neilson

Preface: Introducing the Issues

Introduction

The *Third International Conference* on *Strategic Issues in Health Care Management* took place in St Andrews in early April 1998. Delegates from over 20 countries heard almost 100 presentations on a diverse range of topics – from the big issues of national health systems reform, to the human problems of developing a patient-focused culture. The rain lashed down outside but nothing could dampen the enthusiasm of those tackling the perennial issues of managing quality and controlling costs in health services.

The result of those three days was not only new friends and expanding professional networks, but also two eclectic collections of papers on the twin themes of costs and quality. The papers in this volume, selected from over 80 original high quality submissions, reflect the upsurge of innovative work currently taking place on *managing quality*. Papers in a companion volume examine macro health care reform and micro methods of cost-effectiveness analysis (*Controlling Costs: Strategic Issues in Health Care Management*, Ashgate, 1999).

Scene Setting

The first two chapters in this collection examine the big picture. John Deffenbaugh goes back to first principles to ask whether health care is indeed a business and, if so, what are the implications of this for health care policy and management. To give away the answer to these intriguing questions at this point would be to spoil a skilfully woven story.

Moira Fischbacher and Arthur Francis then examine some of the design issues facing health services, identifying the importance of clear input from a range of different stakeholders. They draw attention to the highly politicized and contextualized nature of the design process, and make a number of particularly timely observations as (in the United Kingdom) Primary Care Groups and Primary Care Trusts struggle to define their form and function.

Quality in Health Care

It is fitting, after quality took centre stage in the latest UK health care reforms (Secretary of State for Health, 1998a, b), that the first section of this book examines this central topic. The key issues covered are what is quality? and how will we know when we've got it? Mike Walsh, Juan Baeza, Michael Calnan and Mike Hart all take varying looks at these questions. Walsh and Hart emphasize the importance of listening to those who know best (the patients), while Baeza and Calnan nicely expose the potential for conflict as clinicians on either side of the purchaser-provider divide differ in their views of what constitutes high quality care.

More important than knowing what quality is, is knowing how to improve it in everyday care settings. A series of three papers examines the role of various audits in improving quality. Gail Johnston and colleagues identify what gets in the way of effective clinical audit, and go on to suggest a range of managerial responses. Chris Southwick and colleagues provide some detailed advice on drawing-in to the audit process 'difficult to get at' health professionals (in this case, general dental practitioners who, because of their independent contractor status, fall outside of more formal networks aimed at improving quality). Sandra Nutley brings this section to a close by exploring the potential of audits of human resource management (HRM) to contribute to health care quality.

Using Performance Indicators

The second section of this book picks up the quality baton but in a decidedly quantitative fashion. As information technology (IT) grows more sophisticated, more powerful and more pervasive, a sea of data swirls around health services. The question is, can these data be turned into useful information? The 1980s and 1990s saw ever-increasing numbers of performance indicators used to compare across different parts of the service (at one point over 2,500 separate indictors were in use in the NHS (Ham and Woolley, 1996)), but many issues surrounding their effective use remain to be clarified.

Richard Wilson asks some searching questions about the use of Hospital

Episode Statistics (HES) and suggests ways in which these might be made more meaningful. Dissatisfaction with the use of activity measures such as HES have in turn led to a growing interest in health outcomes as being more relevant to assessing health care. Steve Kendrick and colleagues from the Scottish Office chart the rise of the Clinical Resource and Audit Group (CRAG) publications on health outcomes which have led the way in the UK in placing such information into the public domain.

The next two papers take a different perspective in shedding light on performance indicators. Régis Blais and colleagues ask what features managers and clinicians want to see in indicators; whereas Anne Ludbrook and Colin Gordon take a broader look at the context within which managers have to respond to indicators, and discuss the dangers of too much focus on the measured to the neglect of the important.

The final two papers in the book explore the important issue of how indicators might be used to bring about beneficial change. Joanne Lally and Richard Thomson highlight the dilemma of trying to take an open and reflective approach to service quality using the same data that may be used to pass (sometimes less than flattering) judgments. Huw Davies and colleagues then extend this by showing the need for a balanced approach between checking on performance (through measurement and publication of indicators) and trusting that professionals will deliver high performance (driven by internal controls).

Concluding Remarks

Improving health care quality has come to the top of the agenda in many developed nations. These papers demonstrate that for all the activity in both practice and research over the past decade there is still much to be done. Managing quality remains a subtle activity with many pitfalls. However, we have learnt much: the terrain is now much more clearly mapped, some unproductive routes have been thoroughly explored and sign-posted, while other roads promise real progress. We hope that you enjoy these contributions, and we look forward to welcoming you to SIHCM 2000* (again in St Andrews) to assess progress on the quality agenda as we enter the next millennium.

Huw T.O. Davies, Manouche Tavakoli
Mo Malek, Aileen R. Neilson
Department of Management, University of St Andrews, Scotland

* For further information on SIHCM 2000 please email SIHCM@st-and.ac.uk.

References

Ham, C. and Woolley, M. (1996), *How Does the NHS Measure Up? Assessing the performance of health authorities*, National Association of Health Authorities and Trusts, Birmingham.

Secretary of State for Health (1998a), *A First Class Service: Quality in the new NHS*, Department of Health, London.

Secretary of State for Health (1998b), *The New NHS: Modern, Dependable*, HMSO, London.

SECTION 1
SCENE SETTING

1 Is Health Care a Business? An Analysis of Health Care, and its Consideration as a Business

JOHN L. DEFFENBAUGH
Frontline Management Consultants

Introduction

This question is now more pertinent than ever in the UK, as the public sector component of the health care industry moves from being structured as a competitive internal market to a format based on cooperation among organizations.

The National Health Service (NHS) was structured as an internal market beginning in 1989 (Secretaries of State, 1989b). This 'reformed' structure resulted in:

- separation of purchasers of health care from providers;
- establishment of new organizations such as NHS trusts and GP fundholders;
- an implicit, competitive management style to compete internally for contracts.

Resources for the Conservative reforms which drove the NHS remained limited, and the idea was that the competition among providers would ensure both enhanced cost effective care, and higher quality. However, shortly after these reforms began being implemented, government ministers began to down-play the business and competitive nature of the new structure. These changed views resulted from different managerial and ministerial priorities, and, in one case, the then Minister of State for Health, William Waldegrave, signalled that the language of business had influenced the NHS too much, and that 'the

Managing Quality: Strategic Issues in Health Care Management, H.T.O. Davies, M. Tavakoli, M. Malek, A.R. Neilson (eds), Ashgate Publishing Ltd, 1999.

NHS is not a business, it is a public service and a great one' (Waldegrave, 1990).

This repositioning of the NHS by the Conservatives coincided with Labour's continuing opposition to the internal market, resulting in the publication of its NHS proposals, which focused on moving from competition to cooperation (Labour Party, 1995). Upon assuming power in 1997, the new government quickly moved to reorientate the NHS. Viewed from a Scottish perspective, particularly recognizing the distinctive nature of the NHS in Scotland (NHSiS), and its anticipated relationship to the pending Scottish Parliament, the new government quickly reaffirmed the nature of the NHS as a 'public service' (Galbraith, 1997). The new framework for the NHSiS was introduced through a White Paper that retained the separation of purchasers and providers, but removed the explicit competitive nature of health care provision (Secretary of State for Scotland, 1997).

However, in framing a cooperative and partnership nature to health care provision for the NHS in Scotland, the Scottish Office took firm control of health care objective setting and accountability, and therefore, implicitly, health care delivery. This was presented by indicating that the Management Executive in charge of the NHSiS would be regarded as 'head office', (Secretary of State for Scotland 1997), and that it viewed the 'NHS in Scotland as a 'firm' to be managed, not an industry of competing businesses to be regulated' (Scottish Office, 1997a). Through taking charge, the Management Executive, operating from St Andrew's House in Edinburgh, will set performance indicators (financial and clinical particularly), appoint managers who can deliver its objectives, and manage proactively the whole process of health care delivery; St Andrew's House will therefore provide a clear lead in both setting tasks and governing behaviour.

The above discussion focuses on the NHS, which is too often regarded as standing for 'health care' (Deffenbaugh, 1994a). In taking a step back, however, and answering the question 'Is health care a business?', it is essential first to address the concept of health care, leading on to an assessment of its nature as a business. The following sections present the analysis in this order.

Health Care

How health care is described depends on where one is sitting, and what is viewed through the window:

- viewed from the NHS, health care is considered to be the delivery of services to patients; while
- viewed from industry, health care is thought of as the manufacturing of products and the delivery of services ultimately to be used by patients and the wider public.

Rather than viewing health care through a window on the ground, the following discussion goes five miles up and considers the concept of health care from a strategic and holistic perspective. The vehicle for this analysis is what is called the 'health care continuum' (Deffenbaugh, 1994a).

The health care continuum, illustrated in Figure 1.1, represents a holistic view of health care, recognizing the impact of the following discreet, yet interlinked, stages on each other: research and development, manufacturing, distribution, and delivery. For each of these functions, there are a number of suppliers; support activities also impact on each area. The stages of the health care continuum are discussed in turn below.

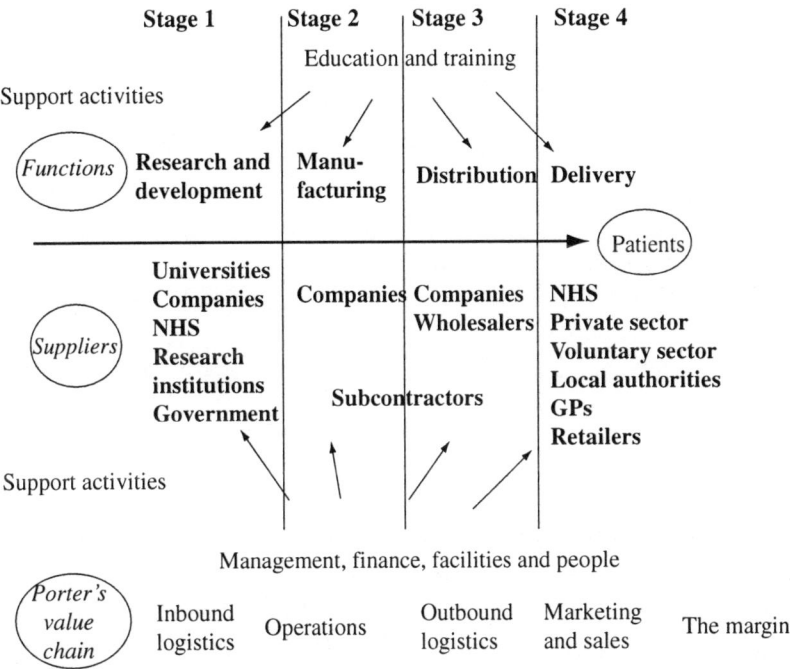

Figure 1.1 Health care continuum

Stage 1 – Research and Development

Players in the research and development (R&D) stage include companies, universities, research institutions, the NHS and government departments. R&D provides the foundation for new product development, and underpins the shape and structure through which health care will ultimately be delivered to patients. The fundamental basis for research and development is indicated by the level of expenditure in the pharmaceutical industry, which, as the *Financial Times* commented on the proposed SmithKline Beecham and American Home Products merger, 'It's the research, stupid' ('Lex' column, 1998).

The fundamental importance of R&D is indicated by the level of this expenditure in the pharmaceutical and health care industries. Table 1.1 below from the *UK R&D Scoreboard* (DTI, 1997) presents the comparison of UK to international R&D in these industries.

Table 1.1   R&D/sales ratios (%)

Sector	UK	International
Health care	3.7	11.3
Pharmaceuticals	12.0	12.2

While the UK compares favourably in pharmaceuticals, it lags dramatically in health care. The annual *R&D Scoreboard*, published by the UK Department of Trade and Industry (DTI) since 1991, shows that average spending on R&D by the world's largest industrial companies (including defence and pharmaceutical companies) has remained steady at about 4.4 per cent of sales, but the UK overall is only 2.3 per cent.

The close linkage of R&D to patient care is now recognized by the NHS, resulting in the production of the *Research and Development Strategy for the NHS in Scotland* (Chief Scientist Office, 1993). Universities and NHS hospitals, in partnership, must now 'earn' research and development funds, through focusing on the outcome of R&D expenditure, which currently amounts to £38.5m in the NHSiS – £28m goes to trusts to support recurring funding, and £10m goes towards health research grants, mainly to universities. The emphasis is increasingly to translate R&D from 'bench to bedside', and this has been reinforced through the recent White Paper by establishing the Scottish Health Technology Assessment Centre (Secretary of State for Scotland, 1997).

A tangible example of the linkage between R&D in academia and the delivery of patient care at the bedside is the establishment of the Clinical Research Facility (CRF) in Edinburgh, with the main facility based at the city's Western General Hospital. Supported by a £4m grant to the University of Edinburgh from the Wellcome Trust, the CRF will conduct patient-focused clinical research into a range of common diseases, including cancer, diabetes and stroke illnesses.

A further dimension of R&D is the trend towards commercialization of research and new product investigations from academia into business. The drivers within academia include the aim to attract commercial funding, but also to provide an output for R&D that is not carried out for the sole purpose of research alone. The drivers for industry are to ensure a stream of new products and processes which underpins the commercial viability of businesses.

In a macroeconomic sense, the benefits of R&D and commercialization are recognized by Scottish Enterprise through its emphasis to grow the economy via new company formation. Spin-outs from academia, often based on commercialization of R&D, will play a key part in enhancing business birth rate in Scotland (McVey, 1996).

The case can therefore be made for research and development as the first stage of the health care continuum, without which manufacturing will be constrained and uncompetitive.

Stage 2 – Manufacturing

This is the second stage of the health care continuum and results from R&D to produce a steady stream of new and creative products and processes. However, the market is very discerning, and very unforgiving of manufactured products that do not meet customer requirements, so the link must therefore be very strong from R&D through manufacturing to ultimate consumption. This is nothing new – as Adam Smith indicated, 'consumption is the sole and purpose of production' (Smith, 1776).

The health care manufacturing sector comprises companies in a number of fields: pharmaceutical, biomedical, bioengineering, medical equipment, biotechnology, disposables, etc. These manufacturers, largely in the private sector in the UK, will in some cases manufacture end products themselves, or form part of a supply chain process resulting in end product manufacturing. Across the UK, the profile of companies (Dun & Bradstreet, 1998) is towards the small and medium-sized enterprise (SME) end of the spectrum – sales of less than £15m – as illustrated in Table 1.2.

Table 1.2   Manufacturing companies in the UK

Sales (£)	No.	%
< 15m	25,864	88.6
15m–30m	1,566	5.4
30m–60m	836	2.9
60m–90m	305	1.0
>90m	605	2.1
Total	**29,176**	**100.0**

Within Scotland, the manufacturing sector overall accounts for 7.5 per cent of VAT-based enterprises, while for England the figure is 9.9 per cent (Office for National Statistics, 1996). Health industry enterprises account for only .53 per cent of the overall businesses in Scotland, and .57 per cent in England. The manufacturing and health care sectors in Scotland are underdeveloped, which reinforces the strong business relationship among not only various parts of the UK, but also within Europe and worldwide.

It is not only products which are 'manufactured', but also services, and these are also included in Stage 2 of the health care continuum. The financial and business services sector alone accounts for 20 per cent of Scottish gross domestic product, compared to 18 per cent for manufacturing (Scottish Office, 1997b). The availability and extent of services equally provides an outlet for R&D, such as with computer information systems and manufacturing processes.

A further dimension to manufacturing, linking this stage of the continuum to support activities, is the 'manufacturing' of specialist skills embodied in the roles of scientists, doctors and others. While education and training is a resource which allows each stage of the continuum to be carried out, the development of skills and expertise in specialist areas is fundamental to the growth and development of health care. Regarded in this way, academic institutions are analogous to companies in manufacturing a 'product'.

Viewed holistically, the manufacturing stage of the health care continuum is fundamental both to providing an output for R&D and to impacting on the way health care is ultimately delivered to patients.

Stage 3 – Distribution

This stage of the health care continuum is where value can be added and/or cost reduced. Michael Porter's value chain (Porter, 1985) indicates how competitiveness can be enhanced through analysing processes to enhance value. From this overview, Figure 1.1 also illustrates the link of the health care continuum itself to the concept of the value chain. The health care industry as a whole can be seen to operate in a similar way to that of an organization, aiming to add value across the length of the continuum.

The distribution stage of the continuum is taking on increased importance in achieving this objective. Both management expertise and financial resources from the private sector are being called upon to enhance public sector services, with the focus on improving health care for patients and the general public. Players in this stage reach back into manufacturing, and forward into delivery, in order to add to the delivery of products and services to end users. Private sector logistics companies contribute scheduling, 'just in time' delivery and inventory expertise to both their private and public sector partners. The acquisition by Unichem of Alliance Sante illustrates the added value and enhanced profitability that exists in this sector.

In marketing terms, this is the 'place' of the four Ps of the marketing mix (Borden, 1964). Effective distribution channels can ensure best fit between manufacturers' products and users' requirements. Innovative and creative approaches to distribution tend to lower organizational boundaries, as logistics companies backwardly integrate into manufacturing premises, and then integrate forward into delivery organizations such as hospitals. Through a partnership approach and commitment to shared working and shared risk, around what are called 'relational contracts' (Kay, 1993), skill and expertise, and in some cases people themselves, can be transferred between organizations. The result can often be learning partnerships, though it must be recognized that the long term aim for the private sector is sustainable competitive advantage and profitability, while the public sector will be seeking to reduce costs, enhance quality and more effectively maximize the use of limited resources.

Stage 4 – Delivery

The above points logically make the link to Stage 4 of the health care continuum, namely the delivery of goods and services to patients and the general public. It is the delivery of hospital and community health services, in tandem with primary care, which is often seen as 'health care' (Deffenbaugh, 1994). While the NHS in Scotland has an expenditure of £4.4b, the reality, however, is that health care *delivery* is only one part of health care, at the final stage of the continuum. The position of general practitioners (GPs) as the 'gatekeepers' of the NHS recognizes their position through which patient care is channelled in the first instance. This pivotal position is reinforced by the support of other players at this stage of the continuum, particularly the public and private hospital sectors and pharmaceutical companies.

In addition to the NHS and its general practitioners, other players in the delivery of health care include the private health care sector (hospitals and nursing homes), pharmacists, retailers, social workers, and the voluntary sector. This mix illustrates the blurred edges between health care and social care, and with the policies of the new government, there is a greater recognition of the link between ill health and the causes of ill health, such as poor housing, lack of employment opportunities, and social deprivation (Secretary of State for Scotland, 1997). The economic impact of the delivery aspects of health care overall, particularly the National Health Service, is illustrated in recent studies by Cogent Strategies International of health care clusters in areas such as Inverness (Cogent, 1996). This work illustrates the links of manufacturing and services to health care delivery, and the potential for economic growth through enhancing the cluster.

The changing dynamics within Stage 4 of the health care continuum are illustrated by the new structural proposals for providers in *Designed to Care* (Secretary of State for Scotland, 1997). On the one hand, the private sector is now being marginalized as a player in the delivery of health care in partnership with the NHS – but not for the financing of assets through the Private Finance Initiative (PFI) – while on the other hand, general practitioners – traditional SMEs – are brought to the fore through the structures of 'primary care trusts' (PCTs) and 'local health care cooperatives' (LHCCs).

Whatever the balance of power among providers, the trend of the spectrum of care (Deffenbaugh, 1994), as illustrated in Figure 1.2, is very much towards shifting resources from institutions to the community.

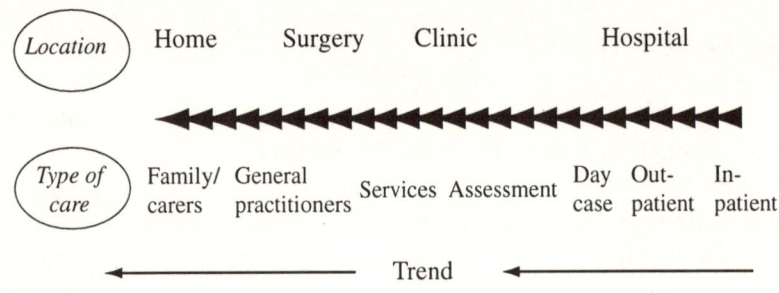

Figure 1.2   Spectrum of care

The drivers of this shift include reducing cost, enhancing quality, encouraging responsibility among users, and enhancing voluntary services and, to a degree, private sector provision. While the NHS will remain a public service, it is apparent that the voluntary sector will not be excluded from playing a significant role in providing these services. It will be interesting, however, to see if proposals to involve the 'independent/private' sector in the provision of community care put forward by the last government (Secretaries of State, 1989b), are continued by Labour ministers.

As the balance of health care provision is shifted within Stage 4 of the continuum, so the use of resources will also change. The key resource areas – people, assets and finance (Ohmae, 1982) – will be significantly impacted through this shift, as illustrated by the continuum:

- people – the types of staff and skill mix providing health care will change, for example the increase in nurse practitioners in primary care;
- assets – the reduced requirement for major fixed asset facilities, such as large hospitals, will significantly impact on proposals for a number of the major PFI hospital projects;
- finance – the requirement to ensure value for money, or 'best value', through the use of financial resources, which also underpins people and asset utilization.

The one certain factor in this equation will be the continuing limited availability of public sector resources to finance health care delivery within Stage 4 of the continuum. Hence, there is the need to closely interlink all the health care activities along the continuum to focus on improving health for individuals and the population overall within limited resources.

This, then, is 'health care'. In concluding this first section, some key points should be made:

- while each stage of the continuum can, to a degree, be viewed discreetly, it is apparent that real added value comes from recognizing and maximizing the linkages within each stage and along the whole continuum;
- the continuously changing range of players within and among each stage offers opportunities to focus on adding value and reducing costs for the benefit of patients and the general public;
- innovations in new technologies, products and services can be seen to have a direct impact upon health care among patients and the general public;
- new processes at each stage can also be seen to have such a direct impact;

- an implicit feedback loop ensures that activities in each stage build on progress from the previous, while at the same time influence results from earlier stages.

If this is 'health care', is it, however, a business?

Business

'"Would you tell me, please", said Alice, "which way I ought to go from here?" "That depends a good deal on where you want to get to", said the Cat' (Carroll, 1865). The point of this paper is to assess health care as a business, and the chosen point of departure has been the health care continuum. The case has been presented that while discreet segments of the continuum can be analysed in their own right, health care from a holistic perspective can only be considered by taking the whole continuum into consideration. The stages of the continuum, combining functions, suppliers and support activities, are integrated and interrelated.

It is time, therefore, to take a step back, and consider what is meant by 'business', after which health care and business will be brought back together to answer the question, 'Is health care a business?'.

Defining 'Business'

The literature most often analyses the meaning of 'business' from the following perspectives:

- 'what business are we in?'; or
- 'what is our business?'; rather than
- 'what is a business?'.

Taking the first question, Theodore Levitt used the example of the American railroad industry to famously highlight the danger of choosing too narrow a definition of the business area in which a company operates (Levitt, 1960). It is not just the private sector which agonizes over what business it is in, but also the public sector – the problems in clarifying the roles of health care and social care illustrate this point, while the NHS as an organization also faces this dilemma (Eskin, 1992).

The second question overlaps with the first, and focuses on business definition in terms of the fit between company resources and market requirements. Defining the business in which an organization operates can conceptually be viewed from three dimensions (Abell, 1980):

- customer groups describe categories of who is being satisfied;
- customer functions describe customer needs, or what is being satisfied;
- technology scope describes the way, or how, customer needs are satisfied.

The question of business definition would also take us into an assessment of business systems, processes and organizations, but it would be too easy to get sidetracked into a discussion about the first two questions, rather than focusing on the third, namely 'what is *a business*?'. This question, however, is seldom addressed in the literature, so let us turn first to *Webster's Dictionary* to establish a baseline: 'business – purposeful activity; activity directed toward some end'. This is broad enough, but goes to one extreme, and is therefore too broad.

In the search for a middle ground, other writers such as Charles Handy (1994, p. 129) comment that

> we are all 'in business' these days, be we doctor or priest, professor or charity-worker. *Every* organization is, in practice, a business, because it is judged by its effectiveness in turning inputs into outputs for its customers or clients, and is judged in competition among its peers. The only difference is that the 'social businesses' do not distribute their surpluses.

The Dean of business writers, Peter Drucker, states that 'in a business, there is a financial bottom line' (Drucker, 1990, p. 81), but he departs from Handy, when discussing 'non-profit organizations', by indicating that 'they are not businesses'. While Drucker views businesses as supplying either goods or services, he regards a non-profit organization as having a 'product' of a 'changed human being'; such organizations are 'human-change agents'. As Drucker states, 'after all, they do not have a 'bottom line''. However, try telling this to the finance director of a non-profit organization, such as an NHS trust, university, or economic development agency, which has to struggle to break even on an annual basis.

Taking the search for the definition of a 'business' further, a useful port of call is the literature on business ethics. This extension of the analysis raises a further question:

- 'what is business for?'.

The ethical debate focuses on this question, resulting in some of the features of business activity highlighted to include its economic character and its conduct in organizations (Boatright, 1993). A business can also be viewed as a 'feedback system' (Sherwin, 1983), with capital owners, employees, and consumers members of the system, all of whom co-produce the output. The purpose of the business for each is as follows:

- owners – yield profits and appreciation of capital;
- employees – afford a living;
- customers – furnishing them with goods and services.

Against this background, it is time to pull these threads together into a strand of criteria that can be used to define a business. The following criteria of a business will therefore be used ultimately to bring health care and business together:

- financial bottom line;
- focus on an end;
- use inputs to product outputs;
- feedback loop from user back to supplier.

A 'business' implies finance, so the first criterion is financial. The other criteria focus on the business 'system', in a similar way to which we have addressed the health care system through the continuum. Having identified criteria for a business, it will be beneficial first to compare and contrast private and public sector views of business, prior to bringing business and health care back together.

Private and Public Sectors

The health care continuum comprises both the public and private sectors, and while together on the continuum, they can be viewed separately. Some of the contrasts are legal and statutory: private companies governed by the various Companies Acts, reporting profits/losses via a profit and loss account (P&L), while public sector organizations report via income and expenditure accounts (I&E). The middle ground, increasingly recognized as the 'social economy', comprises a range of services which help to grow and sustain a community over the long term, such as credit unions, child care provision, community care provision, and local training initiatives for the unemployed. While neither private sector nor public sector, these social economy organizations are largely in the hands of the local community, which both manages and uses these services. Support funding comes largely from the public sector to get these organizations off the ground.

While the private sector, implicitly and explicitly, meets the criteria presented above for 'a business', the position of the public sector is more problematic. The trend in the 1980s and 1990s has been to commercialize the public sector (Deffenbaugh, 1994b), and a number of themes of business became apparent: customer orientation, competition, purchaser/provider framework, contract mechanism, performance targets, and business plans. These and other examples of business terminology entered everyday language in the public sector, such as vision, mission, and corporate strategies. The movement to reinvent government gathered steam with the publication of the book by the same name (Osborne and Gaebler, 1992), which described the principles around which entrepreneurial public organizations operate, such as being mission driven, and encouraging competition.

While there were areas of convergence between the public and private sectors during the Conservative years of government, it also became apparent that the ethos of the public sector could not, and should not, be aligned totally with that of the private sector. The serious financial and administrative failures in public bodies highlighted to the Committee of Public Accounts prompted the committee to prepare a 'checklist of points which public bodies need to keep in mind in order to guard against the risk of such lapses in the proper conduct of public business' (Committee of Public Accounts, 1994).

While the public sector adopted the terminology of the private sector, it did not recognize the real meaning of many of the terms. A good example was in the area of contracting in the purchaser/provider relationship, which became a 'them and us', 'win-lose' battle in the classical contract sense, rather than moving toward a 'win-win', relational contract approach (Kay, 1993). The values of the public sector thus became neglected as overzealous public sector managers, particularly in the NHS, moved to implement what they perceived as business concepts in a manner which would have been anathema to many businessmen themselves (Stewart and Walsh, 1992).

Health Care as a Business

It is time to bring the strands of health care and business together, to answer the question, 'is health care a business?' This question should now be considered against the background of both the earlier definition of health care and the criteria of a business. The answer is yes: the interrelated set of businesses along the continuum seek to add value to the health of the ultimate recipient, so there is a financial bottom line within which inputs are used to the end of health gain, feeding back continuously to earlier stages on the continuum.

Some may not be persuaded by this leap of logic, so let us consider the position of the NHS aspect of health care on its own.

- Does it have a financial bottom line? Yes, to break even annually on income and expenditure, keep within an agreed borrowing limit, and achieve a 6 per cent return on assets.
- Does it focus on an end? Yes, to improve health of the individual and society overall.
- Does it use inputs to achieve outputs? Yes, in the best tradition of Donabedian (Donabedian, 1966).
- Is there a feedback loop from user back to supplier? Yes, particularly in R&D and the bedside training of medical students.

The answer for the NHS is therefore also 'yes'. We will find that the Scottish Office increasingly manages the NHSiS as a business, as it takes central control to direct the use of limited resources to achieve health gain, equity, and clinical objectives. All the indications from *Designed to Care* support this assertion.

Conclusion

Health care is of such critical importance to society, that the subject deserves to be viewed from a holistic perspective – not just the perspective of the beneficiary, but also from the perspectives of the stakeholders in each and every stage of the continuum of health care. Economic benefit is created by both healthy individuals, and healthy companies and organizations, private and public sector. By viewing the question of health care as *a business*, the argument has been placed in a different box from the usual questions about business strategy.

The case has been argued for health care having a meaning that is outside the conventional view of the NHS. The health care continuum does for health care what Michael Porter does via the value chain for an organization. Only by maximizing the relationships along the breadth and depth of the continuum can ultimate value be added to the health of the nation.

The case has also been argued for business to be view against certain criteria. These criteria are broad, and reflect a view from the 1990s, rather than earlier decades. Multi-organization relationships across previous boundaries are beginning to product benefits, and in many cases are a prerequisite of the ability to deliver benefits, such as when applying R&D, or delivering care in the community.

Brought together, health care is, therefore, a business. Following on from this conclusion, the strategic implications for health policy makers and health care managers will be as follows:

- organizations will in future be driven to work across traditional barriers that have defined spheres of influence; in taking a holistic approach to defining what business they are in, companies will find that a partnership route offers the best way of securing sustainable competitive advantage;
- backward or forward integration along the continuum need not, however, be solely by merger or joint venture; rather, outsourcing, subcontracting and relational working could form the basis for achieving the critical mass and synergy that managers will be searching for;
- the drive to reduce costs and improve quality will be enhanced further by working in association with suppliers and buyers in a 'win-win' partnership; this is a lesson well appreciated by the private sector, but only beginning to be learned by the public sector;
- influencing the customer, or patient, will be fundamental to making the best use of health care resources; again, the private sector appreciates this, but the public sector must proactively tackle the insatiable demand on resources through working with patients and the public to control demand;
- finally, public/private partnerships will be more commonplace, not just in areas such as PFI, but also in service provision.

As a business, health care affects all members of society. It is ironic, therefore, that as the last Conservative government tried unsuccessfully to organize and manage health care along business lines, it appears that it will be this Labour government that offers real opportunities for the private sector to work in partnership with the public sector to enhance health care delivery.

References

Abell, D.F. (1980), *Defining the Business*, Prentice-Hall, London.

Borden, N.H. (1964), 'The concept of The Marketing Mix', *Journal of Advertising Research*, June, pp. 2–7.

Chief Scientist Office (1993), *Research and Development Strategy for the National Health Service in Scotland*, The Scottish Office Home and Health Department, Edinburgh.

Cogent Strategies International (1996), *Inverness Health Cluster* (transcript).

Committee of Public Accounts (1994), *The Proper Conduct of Public Business*, House of Commons, HMSO, London.

Deffenbaugh, J. (1994a), 'Health Care Continuum', *Health Manpower Management*, 20 (3), pp. 37–9.

Deffenbaugh, J. (1994b), 'Working to a business agenda', *Public Sector Yearbook 1994*, Insider Publications Ltd, Edinburgh.

Department of Trade and Industry (DTI) (1997), *The UK R&D Scoreboard 1997*, DTI, London.

Donabedian, A. (1966), 'Evaluating the quality of medical care', *Millbank Memorial Federation of Quality*, XLIV, 3, Part 2, pp. 166–203.

Drucker, P. (1992), *Managing the Non-Profit Organisation*, Butterworth-Heinemann, Oxford.

Dun & Bradstreet (1998), *European Dun's Market Identifiers*, Dun & Bradstreet, London.

Eskin, F. (1992), 'What business is the NHS in?', *Journal of Management in Medicine*, 6 (1), pp. 35–43.

Galbraith, S. (1997), *Ministerial Address to Scottish Health Service Conference*, 30 May (transcript).

Handy, C. (1994), *The Empty Raincoat*, Random House, London.

Kay, J. (1993), *Foundations of Corporate Success*, Oxford University Press, Oxford.

Labour Party (1995), *Renewing the NHS*, The Labour Party, London.

Levitt, T. (1960), 'Marketing Myopia' in *Levitt on Marketing, Harvard Business Review, 1987*, Harvard Business School, Boston.

Lex column (1998), 'Research Riches', *Financial Times*, 21 January, p. 22.

McVey, B. (1996), *The Business Birth Rate Strategy Update*, Scottish Enterprise, Glasgow.

Office for National Statistics (1996), *Size Analysis of UK Businesses*, The Stationery Office, London.

Ohmae, K. (1982), *The Mind of the Strategist*, McGraw–Hill, New York.

Osborne, D. and Gaebler, T. (1992), *Reinventing Government*, Addison-Wesley, New York.

Porter, M.E. (1985), *Competitive Advantage*, The Free Press, New York.

Scottish Office (1997a), *Designed to Care* (summary transcript).

Scottish Office (1997b), *The Scottish Abstract of Statistics*, HMSO, Edinburgh.

Secretaries of State for Health, Social Security, Wales, and Scotland (1989a), *Caring for People*, HMSO, London.

Secretaries of State for Health, Wales, Northern Ireland and Scotland (1989b), *Working for Patients*, HMSO, London.

Secretary of State for Scotland (1997), *Designed to Care*, The Scottish Office Department of Health, Edinburgh.

Sherwin, D.S. (1983), 'The ethical roots of the business system' in *The Business of Ethics and Business, Harvard Business Review, 1987*, Harvard Business School, Boston.

Smith, A. (1776), *Wealth of Nations*, currently published by Penguin Books, London.

Stewart, J. and Walsh, K. (1992), 'Change in the management of public services', *Public Administration*, 70, Winter, pp. 499–518.

Waldegrave, W. (1990), *Trafford Memorial Lecture*, Royal College of Surgeons, 12 December (transcript).

2 Managing the Design of Health Care Services

MOIRA FISCHBACHER[1] AND ARTHUR FRANCIS[2]

1 Department of Management Studies, University of Glasgow Business School
2 University of Bradford Management Centre

Introduction

In recent years, considerable attention has been given to the management of product development, particularly within management and engineering disciplines (Hollins and Pugh, 1990; Womack et al., 1990; Brown and Eisenhardt, 1995; Cooper, 1996). Within the field of strategic management, the importance of new product development (NPD) and innovation has increasingly been recognized (Jenkins et al., 1997) as has the interrelatedness of the NPD and innovation process with organizational conditions (see for example Nohria and Gulati 1996). Amabile et al. (1996) wrote:

> Successful implementation of new programs, new product introductions, or new services depends on a person or a team having a good idea – and developing that idea beyond its initial state ... we assume that the social environment can influence both the level and the frequency of creative behaviour ... creativity by individuals and teams is a starting point for innovation ... Creativity is the seed of all innovation, and psychological perceptions of innovation ... within an organization are likely to impact the motivation to generate new ideas.

Furthermore, innovation is not only seen as a means of gaining competitive advantage but as a 'primary means for corporate renewal' (Dougherty, 1992).

Theoretical developments around NPD/design (terms which we use interchangeably) and innovation have mainly been from manufacturing research. Surprisingly little research has been on product development in the service sector despite the fact that in Great Britain the service sector accounts for 50 per cent of GDP (Wisemewski, 1997) and 75 per cent of employment

Managing Quality: Strategic Issues in Health Care Management, H.T.O. Davies, M. Tavakoli, M. Malek, A.R. Neilson (eds), Ashgate Publishing Ltd, 1999.

(compared to manufacturing's 22 per cent and 18 per cent respectively) (Office for National Statistics, 1996).

Design – Context and Meaning

The lack of interest in health service design is somewhat surprising. Although there is no market as in manufacturing, the existence of consumers is undisputed. Furthermore, efforts to produce quality services focused on the consumer (patient) have increased in recent years. A number of hospitals in the UK have adopted and adapted philosophies such as patient focused care (PFC) and the named nurse, attempting to focus on the patient and on quality (Taylor, 1996) in a climate of consumerism which has been stimulated by initiatives like the Patients' Charter and an emphasis on citizens' rights. Coupled with financial pressures on all health service providers to reduce their costs and improve their organizational efficiency, attention to service delivery is merited.

Health Authorities (HAs) and hospitals are faced with the reality of design to an increasing extent. It is interesting to note that the December 1997 White Paper on the NHS in Scotland was entitled *Designed to Care* (The Scottish Office Department of Health 1997). In a climate which stresses a move towards evidence-based medicine, efficient services and customization, how does one go about conceptualizing, for example, an ambulatory care centre? How does one translate the concept into an articulated service idea, gain the support and ownership of the health care professionals who are to deliver the service, design the building, decide upon staffing levels and skills mix, consider the health service process experienced by the patients and so on? Added to that, how can this be done in a way which meets the needs and/or desires (the criteria) of patients, carers, GPs, hospitals and health authorities, to mention only a few of the potential stakeholders? Clearly such a task involves a number of people with appropriate skills, experience and knowledge to address the components of the overall service.

The Nature of Services – What is Being Designed

Service sector products are more complex than manufactured products. Services are intangible and heterogeneous, and are delivered and consumed simultaneously (Zeithaml et al., 1990; Ennew et al., 1995). The spectrum ranges from services with a large tangible component to those with a little or none. Chase and Tansik (1983) identify three types of service: pure, mixed and quasi-manufacturing. Pure services are carried out in the presence of the customers and include medical care. Mixed services involve a combination of face-to-face contact and back office work (e.g. a bank branch). Quasi-manufacturing services involve virtually no face-to-face contact (e.g. distribution centres, ATM financial services).

Pure services rely heavily on customer involvement with the service provider. Their heterogeneity is because service quality is dependent on the quality of the personnel delivering it, which increases the potential for variability. Ballantyne et al. (1995) note that 'staff may be blamed for 'service' problems if the internal data processing 'back up' is not supportive. Quality must be built into the *total service system* or variation will be experienced as poor or inconsistent service'. Some service providers have automated the delivery process, for example in financial services and fast food outlets. Although health services are not amenable to large-scale automation, they are amenable to ongoing service delivery improvements.

Process Quality and Product Quality

Developed in the US in the late 1980s and derived from operational research (Garside, 1993), PFC brings elements of process re-engineering and TQM together with multi-skilling and teamwork (Buchan, 1995a) to focus service processes around the consumer. Those who have implemented PFC have claimed quality improvements, increased patient satisfaction, increased job satisfaction for staff, and improved efficiency (Buchan, 1995b). Also attempting to be more customer-focused, some hospitals have embarked upon business process reengineering/redesign (BPR) (NHS Executive, 1997). Recent BPR experiences at Leicester Royal Infirmary have claimed considerable benefits in a number of areas:

> We started to track patients through the healthcare process and were horrified at what we saw because hospitals are typically organized by functions or departments rather than by healthcare processes (member of the hospital's Centre for Best Practice (Whyte 1997)).

The Leicester project team considered that between 30 per cent and 70 per cent of hospital work was not adding value to the patient and up to 50 per cent of the patient's process steps involved a stage whereby their file was passed from one person/service to another, the point at which things tended to go wrong. They also concluded that no one was responsible for the patient and had an end-to-end experience. Job roles were fragmented and isolated.

Quality extends beyond the care process though, to include health outcomes – the result of the procedure or treatment. Parasuraman et al. (cited in Ennew et al., 1995) suggest there are two aspects of service quality: technical quality and functional quality. Technical quality refers to the extent to which a product (e.g. a surgical procedure) conforms to specifications (i.e. clinical care) whilst functional quality refers to the way in which the service is delivered (i.e. care management). The quality of the service depends, therefore, on the systems in place to treat the patient and the skills of the health care practitioners/ service providers. Clearly, when developing a service, one needs to consider the technical skills of those delivering the service, the technical quality of the procedure/treatment and the functional quality of the process which takes the patient from admission to discharge bearing in mind the service is largely intangible and the product of considerable professional judgment.

Models of Design

There are a number of models for NPD. They build on a 1982 model (Booz, 1982) and have been modified to speed up and improve the quality of the NPD process (Cooper, 1996; Jenkins et al., 1997). They typically identify distinct stages and points at which particular decisions must be made. (The stage-gate model, a typical NPD model, is shown in Figure 2.1). Some models have been carried over into the service sector (Booz, 1982; Hollins and Hollins, 1991; Ennew et al., 1995) but with little adaptation to the service sector context. Where it has been given, attention to service sector NPD has generally been within financial services (Scheuing and Johnson, 1989; Storey and Easingwood, 1993; Edgett, 1996).

The models provide a systematic approach to NPD but, like other top-down prescriptive management processes, can be criticized as decontextualized, linear and rational (Mintzberg, 1990). As Maffin et al. (1997) point out, 'the characteristics of companies and their competitive environments, and their range of strategic and operational choices, are both complex and diverse. As a result, companies may find that interpreting these best practice models in the context of their own circumstances represents a greater challenge today than in the past'.

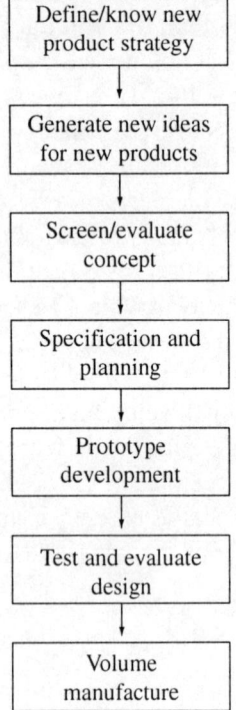

Figure 2.1   A seven stage product development process

Source: Jenkins et al.

- political sensitivity and complexity, e.g. a number of communities with unaligned objectives being subjected to a high number of politically-driven initiatives;
- the diversity of segments (i.e. number of products and services x number of customers): e.g. in a typical acute hospital there are over 4,000 'product lines' provided to many types of 'customer' with many different 'buyers';
- its work being subject to clinical judgment, whereas in the commercial sector the main mechanisms of production do not make resource consuming and quality setting judgments;
- business rules not applying in the same way, as, despite the internal market, different funding principles apply (e.g. the amount of money you have each year is not determined by you but by Government) (NHS Executive 1997).

Figure 2.2   Factors which make the NHS uniquely complex

The NHS has been considered unique because of its 'extra complexity' due to a number of macro and micro level features (see Figure 2.2). Speaking about Leicester Royal Infirmary's redesign, Helen Bevan from their Centre for Best Practice said:

> It took us a long time to understand that the healthcare process is different from the industrial model ... healthcare is unique because of the political complexity which arises from the number of communities involved with unaligned objectives – government, purchasers, general practitioners, internal staff, etc. (Whyte 1997).

The NHS is highly political, comprising a number of professional disciplines with their own agendas, ethics and philosophies and because it delivers a public service paid for through the tax system, it is subject to enormous political intervention. Macro level considerations have a profound impact on the micro level of service delivery and this needs to be considered when services are being designed.

Towards a Service Sector Design Model

In health services the product and the environment are complex, and the design models available do not translate effectively to this sector. Therefore, given the importance of service quality and delivery, we have developed a way of conceptualizing how this process might be managed. Drawing on examples from empirical work carried out between October 1995 and December 1997 and funded by the UK Design Council, this paper demonstrates how the management of service design and service quality is embedded within a social, political, multi-level, multi-organizational process. There are a number of stakeholders in the process each of whom have their own criteria for a well designed service, plus influences external and internal to the organization(s) managing the design (Francis and Fischbacher, 1997).

There are three fundamental relationships in service design (see Figure 2.3). If the designer, having taken a customer perspective, produces a design which is not adopted by the service provider then service quality is jeopardized because the delivered service may not meet the criteria specified by the customer. Alternatively, the service provider may be criticized for providing an unsatisfactory service when the problem is fundamentally one of poor service design.

As O'Connor (1997) notes, 'Patients and public assume that the surgeon

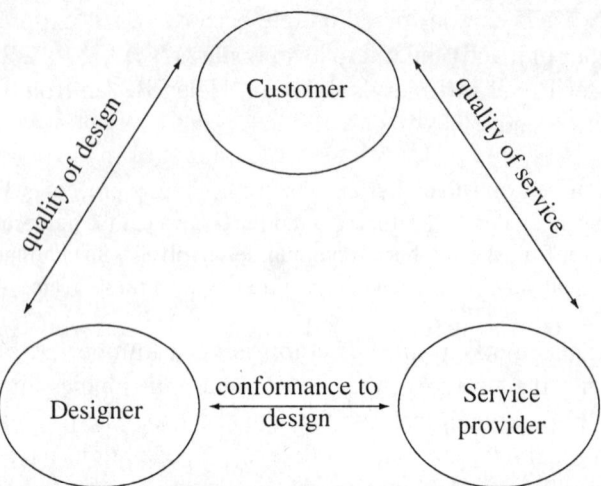

Figure 2.3   Fundamental relationships in design

is responsible for the quality of surgical care and that they are protected from substandard care by quality monitoring conducted by professional bodies'. When clinical care is at an unacceptably poor level, the spotlight is on the clinician even although they may have little control over the outcome:

> These cases occur with some frequency and often concern high visibility specialties with easy-to-count outcomes. Yet causal attribution is difficult since most clinicians provide care in complex settings over which individuals exert only limited control. In cardiac care the skills of the anesthesiologist, perfusionist, cardiac intensive care nurse, and others also affect the outcomes of care (ibid).

This quotation demonstrates service complexity and the difficulties in maintaining service quality. There is also the question of whether what is being delivered is what was intended, i.e., does it conform to the design? Figure 2.3 shows how the relationship between customers and service providers is contingent upon the degree of conformance to and the quality of the design. It also indicates that the designer(s) must have a good understanding of the consumer's perspective if the service is to meet consumer needs.

Managing Design – Empirical Evidence

Our research identified a service design process which spans three organizational levels: macro (strategic), meso (business level) and micro (team/ individual). This paper draws on two case studies: the design of three community mental health resource centres and the design of a community hospital. Both design projects were stimulated by changing policies towards community care and the NHS and Community Care Act 1990. The cases show the stages at which design decisions were made and the emphasis placed upon service delivery.

Case 1: Community Mental Health Resource Centres

Macro level Government legislation deems that a greater proportion of services for mentally ill patients have to be provided within the community. In 1990, one Scottish Health Board (HB) reflected on a history of ongoing research into clinical research, needs assessment, epidemiological studies and mental health assessments and began to think about the idea of providing services from community based resource centres (RCs). RCs are team organizations offering medical, nursing, occupational and other therapeutic services. Based throughout the city, they are accessed mainly via GP referral. The three in this study serve the severely and chronically mentally ill.

Macro level issues were to do with decommissioning existing services in tandem with commissioning new services. Much attention was directed towards the stakeholders and an overall coordinating group was set up (see Figure 2.4). The majority of the work was done in collaboration with the meso level particularly because early design began when the community trust was still a directly managed unit (DMU).

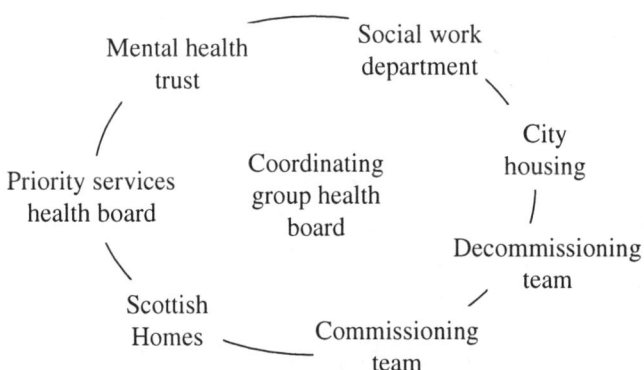

Figure 2.4   Health board coordinating group, macro level

Meso level There are two phases to the meso level design activities. Between 1990 and 1992, an external group of academic consultants advised and managed initial stakeholder liaison, worked on the resource centre concept and facilitated research, training, the ultimate decision-making process and implementation of the early resource centres. The emphasis was on stakeholder days and stakeholder conferences. Interested parties were invited to join discussions about proposed community services although the extent to which this occurred on a large scale diminished as time went on. During discussions, stakeholders were asked about their individual criteria for the centres and the relevant organizations were represented. (For a full account of the generic process taken by the consultancy see Smith, 1995.) The process changed after 1992 and the Trust managed activities themselves following similar principles. Crucial to the RCs' success was support from the medical consultants, so the Trust's Chief Executive dealt directly with them to secure their confidence early on.

Micro level Each RC had to consider three aspects of design: the building, the staffing and the service. Three very different models emerged, despite similar macro and meso influences (see Figure 2.5).

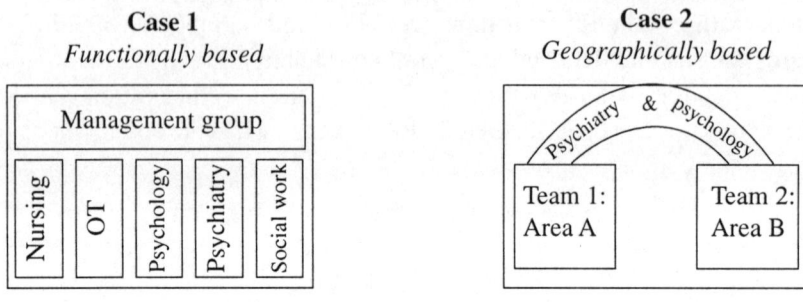

Figure 2.5   Resource centre models

Centre 1. This RC was the product of discussions between practitioners (psychiatrists, community psychiatric nurses (CPNs), GPs, social workers, etc.) within the specific area the centre was to serve. They identified criteria for the location, the building, the way the service would work and integrate with existing community services, and the profile of staff who would make up the RC team. Whilst there was general agreement in most areas, there were some conflicting criteria. GPs wanted a service which made provision for those in immediate distress but this was outwith the RC's criterion of 'severely and chronically mentally ill'. Similarly, the location of the building did not meet all the stakeholders' criteria. The area's geographical characteristics made it difficult to find a suitable location and a subsequent, unrelated event resulted in the trust ultimately securing a building over which the RC had no influence.

Much discussion centred around staffing and service provision. The staffing profile was modelled on an RC elsewhere in the city, comprising a large component of nursing staff, plus some OT, psychology, psychiatry and social work input – a structure similar to a hospital ward. Referrals are made to the team and each week senior members from each discipline meet to decide who should take on the cases. The work tends to be organized according to occupational disciplines.

Centre 2. Initial design work was done in this RC by a small group of health care professionals who had worked in the area for many years, some within a day hospital service. They took the initiative to develop a RC and worked with the Trust put together a business case for Scottish Office funding. This group shared a vision for a small, highly qualified team of multi-disciplinary workers with a smaller nursing input than had been the case in the hospital wards and in other RCs. After some initial work they appointed RC staff who became involved in the design process adding their views and experience. The introduction at a later stage of a number of new employees brought with it the difficulty of continually having to review former decisions and discussions in order to keep new staff fully informed so they could make a meaningful contribution. GPs were not invited to give their criteria but were invited to a meeting at which the RC's raison d'être was explained. Other external stakeholders were involved during the project proposal at a meso level but not at the micro level as in Centre 1.

This RC has the smallest team. Staff work in two sub-teams – one for each of the locations covered by the Centre. The CPN from each sub-team works very closely with the main health centres in the area and tries to attend GP practice meetings. Referrals are made to the sub-teams. The psychiatrist and psychologist however cover both sub-teams so select cases which they need to deal with then the others allocate the remainder between themselves. They try to ensure that sub-teams function in a multidisciplinary way and do so by placing an emphasis on generic assessments of patients. The building design was not an issue because they expanded into existing day hospital facilities.

Centre 3. This RC was principally designed by the consultant psychiatrist who had previously worked in England and came to Scotland with a clear model of how the RC's staffing and processes would be structured. The model was modified to suit the locality. External stakeholders were not invited to suggest how the RC should function but were asked about how the RC should be integrated and any concerns the had were addressed.

The RC is divided into three teams for continuing, community and crisis care. The overall staffing profile is large and makes use of more lower grades of staff e.g., health care assistants, than do the other centres. All the staff discussed and shaped the operational aspects of how each of the mini-teams in the RC would function and formulated team policies. Referrals are made to the member of the team chosen by the GP so there is no group case allocation meeting, only ongoing clinical and business meetings.

Finding a suitable building proved more difficult than in the other two cases. One ideal building was identified but after negotiation with local politicians and town councils, the proposal fell through. Residents were not happy having a mental health centre in their neighbourhood. Some time later, alternative accommodation was found in a local business centre and procured without opposition after considerable efforts to negotiate with and reassure local residents.

Design ideas To an extent the resource centre idea was stimulated during discussions at the interface between the macro and meso levels. The concept, however, finds its origins in America (Dean and Freeman, 1993). It was subsequently adopted in Australia (Hoult, 1990) and then the UK. Initial results of the UK experience were published in the early 1990s (Dean and Gadd, 1990; Dean et al., 1993), by which time the concept had evolved.

Case 2: Community Hospital

Macro level Community care legislation stimulated one Scottish Health Board (HB) to set up a working group (known here as the project board (PB)) to consider alternative service reconfigurations. GP medium acute inpatient, consultant and paramedical outpatient services, day hospital services and other diagnostic and specialist services for the elderly and mentally ill, and the younger (<65) physically disabled were all required for the area.

Key stakeholders in the service (see Figure 2.6) were invited to join the PB which conducted an appraisal of eight service configurations, ranging from minimal changes of existing provision, to split site services and a new single site service. They focused on integrating new and existing services and evaluated the options against the criteria of equity, efficiency, effectiveness, access, choice, comprehensiveness, appropriateness and flexibility. There was no disagreement between PB members as to the suitability of these criteria but complexities still emerged during the scoring:

> 9 out of 11 respondents returned completed forms, five of which were accompanied by written comments explaining the scores given. The remaining two respondents felt that none of the options were appropriate and that written comments would capture the complexities of the arguments for and against the options more adequately than numerical scores. They put forward an alternative option (Official Project Documentation).

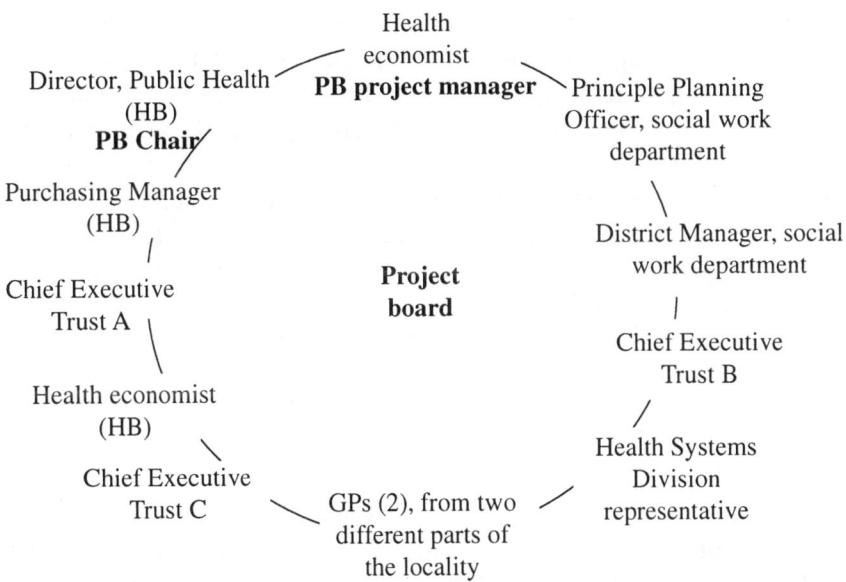

Figure 2.6   Stakeholders in the community hospital design

A single site option in one particular location received the highest score but a lower ranked single site option in an alternative location within the HB area was also considered. Two Trusts, each favouring a different location, declared an interest in providing the services. Prior to issuing an invitation to tender, the PB engaged in a public consultation exercise. Local opinion was so divided that the Trusts organized petitions in support of their proposals and GPs delivered 'campaign' material to homes in the area. Completed tenders had to address the service, building and staffing of the hospital and were evaluated by the PB using a standard investment appraisal methodology.

Meso level The Trust which won the tender had set up a project team (PT) during the public consultation process. PT members included a clinical specialist and personnel from estates and facilities, community services, finance, general practice and the executive. The building design was undertaken by a technical design team (TDT) (architect, quantity surveyor, etc.), who worked closely with the project manager of the PT and with the clinical specialist to design the facilities.

The PT met once or twice each week for updates and to allocate tasks (usually in accordance with individual functional responsibilities). In order to identify cost implications and invite design suggestions, close liaison was maintained with the TDT and with personnel in finance and community services as well as other stakeholders such as consultants, professionals such as paramedics, physiotherapists, etc. (see Figure 2.7). The tender had to be very detailed about building design, staffing profiles and the service process.

Micro level The hospital is yet to be built and so data are not currently available at the micro level. However, the tender documentation includes details about protocols, clinical pathways, supervisory arrangements, grades and job descriptions of staff. The role for multi-skilled generic workers (stewards) whose duties, training schemes and career progression were investigated at length, was included in the design. A clinical development group was then set up to address the admission criteria, training and care protocols prior to staff being employed.

Political environment The political environment was characterized by a divergence of opinion between GPs, local politicians, hospital consultants, Trust hospitals and the general public because many valued the traditional provider and the existing location of services. At the macro level it was felt that one of the major tasks was to keep everybody on board despite the

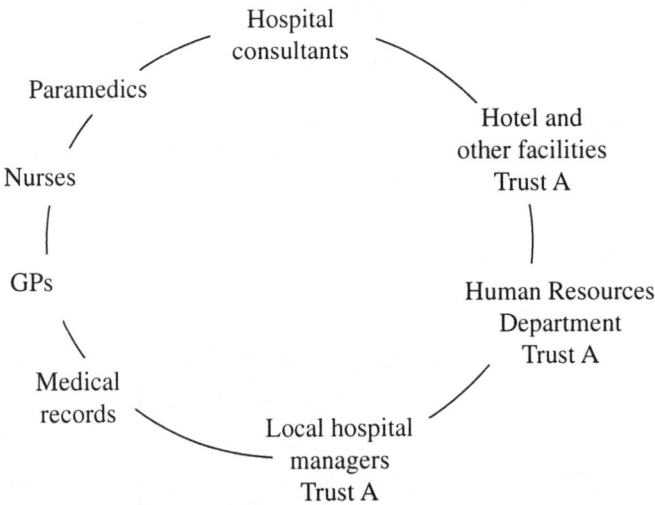

Figure 2.7   Stakeholders in design, the meso level

viewpoints being 'essentially irreconcilable' (PB member) and the potential for resignations by PB members. The Trust felt it necessary to employ a PR consultant to manage relationships with the general public in a campaign involving posters, press conferences and leaflet drops led by the GPs.

Design ideas The design was underpinned by the patient focused care philosophy (PFC). All the physical attributes of the building, staffing and service process needed to suit the patient. This particular design is one of the few facilities in the UK designed entirely on the PFC principle. Other PFC projects are generally implemented in old facilities, single wards or laboratories (Garside, 1993). The ideas then whilst innovative, were adapted from previous PFC sites (including another from within the Trust). Designers deliberately rejected traditional designs (e.g. H-shaped wards, wards with nursing stations) for more economic and effective solutions.

Meeting the Design Challenge: Designing Quality Services

It is clear from the discussion that design in the NHS is complex because of the nature of the service being designed and because of the number of organizations and stakeholders involved. It also transpired during the research that designers need to be able to cope with unanticipated (emergent) factors at all levels (e.g. organizational restructuring, changes in organizational and national policy).

At the macro level the focus is less detailed and broader in scope (see Figure 2.8). Criteria incorporated here are combined and communicated to the meso level where further criteria and stakeholder views are taken into account.

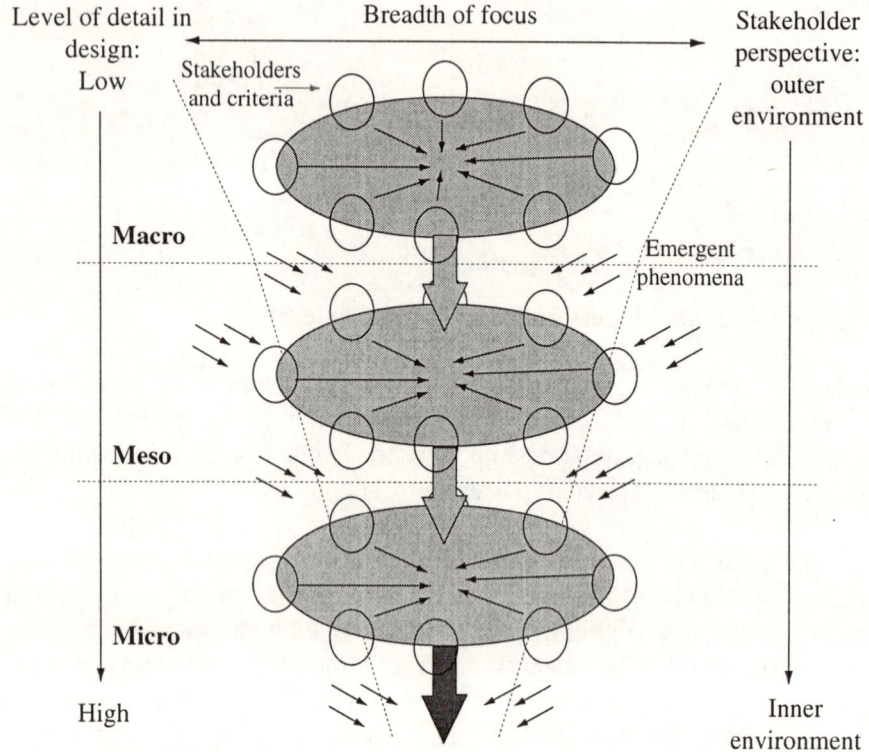

Figure 2.8   The service sector design process

At the micro level service deliverers were, and continue to be, the main focus of the design. In each of the RCs the role of the professions, reporting relationships, degree of generic work and interdisciplinary work took up most of the discussion and it is likely that this will be experienced in the community hospital too. The product itself (the clinical or therapeutic care) was thought to be intuitive to the health care professional delivering it, a 'given' derived from training and experience. It was the mode in which this product would be delivered which attracted attention.

Emergent phenomena (e.g. changing patient needs, new technology, Trust policies, staffing policies) occurred at all stages, even when the service was actually being delivered. A degree of flexibility needed to be allowed so service providers could respond to changing circumstances. Furthermore, when new issues arose they threatened to divert resources (human and financial) away from the design in hand so this tension had to be carefully managed.

The Design Challenge in the New NHS

The framework which has been presented in this paper has many implications for the design of the new primary health care trusts (PHCTs), local health care cooperatives (LHCCs) and primary care groups (PCGs) envisaged for the Scottish and English health services (The Scottish Office Department of Health, 1997; The Department of Health, 1997). The new structures will bring under one organizational umbrella, GPs and community health service providers (e.g. nurses, psychologists, psychiatrists) who will need to work together in a more integrated and formalized fashion than they have in the past. In addition, the new structures mean these groups need to work closely with other organizations to plan and design health care provision across LHCC areas. Stakeholders will include acute trusts, social work departments, voluntary sector providers, health authorities/boards, patients and many others each of whom will have their own, not necessarily convergent, criteria for 'good design'.

At a macro level, health board/authority strategies for developing PHCTs, etc. will need to take cognisance of the multiple stakeholders involved. As shown in Figure 2.2, engaging the service providers in design will prove crucial to the adoption and implementation of new organization and process designs. There are various associations (e.g. local health councils, GP associations) who represent large bodies of stakeholder groups and who could provide valuable input into design. Ignorance, lack of ownership of, or opposition to, designed policies, structures and processes for service provision and administration may result in uncoordinated, poor quality provision.

Health board discussions will be concerned with the broader environment of city-wide service integration but will set the framework for more detailed design so the link between macro, meso and micro criteria and decisions is crucially important. Where possible, there should be cross membership of design teams so that the design and communication process is continuous and as smooth as possible. This will be particularly challenging as meso (PHCT) design will probably be done in parallel with micro (LHCC) level design. The micro level detail, much of which may only become clear as new structures are implemented, will prove particularly important. Organizational arrangements need to be flexible enough to respond to ongoing policy development at regional and national levels, changes in the locality and knowledge acquired as LHCCs/Trusts learn from their experiences. Working relationships will take time to develop and are unlikely to be trouble-free. For example, research has shown that GPs expect to experience difficulties agreeing service priorities across a locality (Fischbacher and Francis, 1998) and staff within the resource centres experienced difficulties when learning to work together in teams because previously they offered parallel services.

The case studies showed how important it is for designers to be clear about what their respective criteria are and to clarify at an early stage, the vision towards which they are working. Resource centre staff, for example, thought they shared an understanding of what a resource centre was. It transpired, however, that their views differed, affecting the philosophies underpinning, for example, the locus of service delivery and relationships with GPs. To assume that all parties have a common understanding about PHCTs, etc. could lead to similar complications. It also became clear during this research that designers need time to design. It is likely that those involved in decisions about PCHTs and LHCCs will have additional responsibilities as part of their ongoing clinical or managerial work and there is a danger that design work may be is set aside, given less attention than it merits. Steps ought to be taken to ensure that design is a priority and that other commitments can be met from additional staffing resources during the design phase.

Finally, organizational transformations take time. Managing the change process and providing training are important elements of design. It is important that designers clarify the nature of new organizational roles and departmental, clinical and decision making boundaries. As new organizational forms are established, there will need to be continual review of service provision if a designed health service is to be realized, but as service provision from health, social and voluntary service organizations differs across any one city, the temptation to draw a detailed blueprint for micro level activities should be avoided.[1]

Note

1   The authors would like to thank the health care professionals from the resource centres and the community Trusts who have supported and contributed to this study both in interviews and during ongoing discussions.

References

Amabile, T.M., Conti, R., Coon, H., Lazenby, J.E. and Herron, M. (1996), 'Assessing the Work Environment for Creativity', *Academy of Management Journal*, 39 (5), pp. 1154–84.

Ballantyne, D., Christopher, M. and Payne, A. (1995), 'Improving the Quality of Services Marketing: Service (Re)design is the Critical Link', *Journal of Marketing Management*, 11 (1/3), pp. 7–24.

Booz, A. and Booz, H. (1982), *New Product Management for the 1980s*, research report.

Brown, S.L. and Eisenhardt, K.M. (1995), 'Product Development – Past Research, Present Findings, and Future-Directions', *Academy of Management Review*, 20 (2), pp. 343–78.

Buchan, J. (1995a), 'Focusing on the Patient?', report for the Management Development Group of the NHS in Scotland.

Buchan, J. (1995b), 'Patient-focus pocus?', *Nursing Management*, 2, 7 November, pp. 6–7.

Chase, R.B. and Tansik, D.A. (1983), 'The Customer Contact Model for Organisation Design', *Management Science*, 29 (9), pp. 1037–50.

Cooper, R.G. (1996), 'Overhauling the New Product Process', *Industrial Marketing Management*, 25 (6), pp. 465–82.

Dean, C. and Freeman, H. (eds) (1993), *Community Mental Health Care: International Perspectives on Making it Happen*, Gaskell & The Centre for Mental Health Services Development, London.

Dean, C. and Gadd, E.M. (1990), 'Home Treatment for Acute Psychiatric Illness', *British Medical Journal*, 301, 3 November, pp. 1021–3.

Dean, C., Phillips, J., Gadd, E.M., Joseph, M. and England, S. (1993), 'Comparison of Community Based Service with Hospital Based Service for People with Acute, Severe Psychiatric Illness', *British Medical Journal*, 307, 21 August, pp. 473–6.

Department of Health (1997), *The New NHS: Modern – Dependable*, White Paper Cm3807, December, The Stationery Office, London.

Dougherty, D. (1992) 'A Practice-Centred Model of Organizational Renewal Through Product Innovation', *Strategic Management Journal*, 13, pp. 77–92.

Edgett, S.J. (1996), 'The New Product Development Process for Commercial Financial Services', *Industrial Marketing Management*, 25 (6), pp. 507–15.

Ennew, C., Watkins, T. and Wright, M. (eds) (1995), *Marketing Financial Services*, 2nd edn, Butterworth Heinemann, Oxford.

Fischbacher, M. and Francis, A. (1999), 'Relationships in Health Care Commissioning', this volume.

Francis, A. and Fischbacher, M. (1997), 'Managing Service Sector Product Design', working paper presented at the British Academy of Management Conference, London.

Garside, P. (1993), 'Patient Focused Care; A Review of Seven Sites in England', report on behalf of the NHSME.

Hollins, B. and Pugh, S. (1990), *Successful Product Design What to do and When*, Butterworths, London.

Hollins, G. and Hollins, B. (1991), *Total Design: Managing the Design Process in the Service Sector*, 1st edn, Pitman Publishing, London.

Hoult, J. (1990), 'Dissemination in New South Wales of the Madison model' in I.M. Marks and R.A. Scott (eds), *Mental Health Care Delivery: Innovations, impediments and implementation*, Cambridge University Press, Cambridge.

Jenkins, S., Forbes, S., Durrani, T.S. and Banerjee, S.K. (1997), 'Managing the Product Development Process – (Part I: an assessment)', *International Journal of Technology Management*, 13 (4), pp. 359–78.

Maffin, D., Thwaites, A., Alderman, N., Braiden, P. and Hills, B. (1997), 'Managing the Product Development Process: Combining Best Practice with Company and Project Contexts', *Technology Analysis and Strategic Management*, 9 (1), pp. 53–74.

Mintzberg, H. (1990), 'The Design School: Reconsidering the Basic Premises of Strategic Management', *Strategic Management Journal*, 11, pp. 171–95.

NHS Executive (1997), *Business Process Reengineering in the NHS*, Ref. No.D4055, edited by P. Crouch.

Nohria, N. and Gulati, R. (1996), 'Is Slack Good or Bad for Innovation?', *Academy of Management Journal*, 39 (5), pp. 1245–64.

O'Connor, G.T. (1997), 'Every System is Designed to Get the Results it Gets', *British Medical Journal*, 315 (7113), pp. 897–8.

Office for National Statistics (1966), 'Table 1.1 Employees in employment: March 1996', *Labour Market Trends*, 104 (8), ss. 12–13.

Scheuing, E.E. and Johnson, E.M. (1989), 'New Product Development and Management in Financial Institutions', *International Journal of Bank Marketing*, 7, pp. 17–21.

Scottish Office Department of Health (1997), *Designed to Care: Renewing the National Health Service in Scotland*, White Paper Cm3811, December 1997, The Stationery Office, Edinburgh.

Smith, H. (1995), 'Strategic Planning of Mental Health Services', *Community Care Management and Planning*, 3, 1 February, pp. 4–11.

Storey, C. and Easingwood, C. (1993), 'The Impact of the New Product Development Project on the Success of Financial Services', *The Service Industries Journal*, 13, pp. 40–54.

Taylor, D. (1996), 'Quality and Professionalism in Health Care: A review of current initiatives in the NHS', *British Medical Journal*, 312, 9 March, pp. 626–9.

Whyte, F. (1997), 'A Big Public Hospital Embarks on Re-engineering', European Commission publication replacing the former *Social Europe Magazine*, *Forum*, 1, October, pp. 19–21.

Wisemewski, D. (ed.) (1997), *Annual Abstract of Statistics*, Office of National Statistics, The Stationery Office, London.

Womack, J.P., Jones, D.T. and Roos, D. (1990), *The Machine that Changed the World*, New York: Rawson Associates, Macmillan Publishing.

Zeithaml, V.A., Parasuraman, A. and Berry, L.L. (1990), *Delivering Service Quality: Balancing customer perceptions and expectations*, The Free Press, New York.

SECTION 2
QUALITY IN HEALTH CARE

3 Towards Critical Quality

MIKE WALSH

Faculty of Health, University of Hull

Introduction

The NHS reforms were the backdrop to the first *strategic issues* conference (St Andrews, 1993). According to Maynard (1992) the role of the consumer was one of the unresolved issues of the 1989 NHS reforms at a time when there was increasing professional consciousness about the importance of consumer judgment. Consequently the Department of Health (1995) commissioned research into the role of consumers in the NHS which led to the *patient partnership* strategy. In 1997 a *patient partnership coordinator* was appointed to oversee this strategy. Why does the NHS need a patient partnership strategy? Quite simply it is because without it the NHS is more likely *to fail badly* to achieve quality. To understand this it is necessary to consider the meaning of quality. Unfortunately, this thinking task is all but absent from virtually *all texts* on quality in health services, or in industry. One way of filling this gap is go back and reconstruct the meaning of quality from the social action viewpoints that Habermas (1991) has set out and analysed in great detail. From this, three perspectives on quality management emerge: *strategic quality*, *normative quality* and *critical quality*. These categories permit us to see easily from a practical but theoretically rigorous viewpoint what the plethora of health service quality initiatives stand for – *patient partnership* included. I will argue that for as long as strategic quality and normative quality continue to dominate the NHS it will face continual reformation. Only *critical quality* offers the possibility that the achievement of quality in the NHS will not recede like the smile on the face of the Cheshire Cat. I will argue that the patient partnership strategy is a step toward critical quality but this can *only* happen if the conditions necessary to achieve critical quality are introduced.

Managing Quality: Strategic Issues in Health Care Management, H.T.O. Davies, M. Tavakoli, M. Malek, A.R. Neilson (eds), Ashgate Publishing Ltd, 1999.

Defining Quality

Despite a long history of quality thinking (see Ellis and Whittington, 1993) it is only in the last quarter of the twentieth century that the concepts and processes of quality management have taken off. This has occurred under the influence of the increasingly long list of so-called *quality gurus*, many of whom provide their own brief definitions of the term 'quality' (for example see Deming, 1982; Crosby, 1984; Juran, 1988; Ishikawa and Lu, 1985). The most widespread definition in commerce and industry is pithily stated by Oakland (1993, p. 4): 'Quality means simply meeting the customers requirements'.

While customer requirements in manufacturing are assumed to be self evident quality in health services, in contrast, has largely been driven by the views of two health service quality 'gurus', Maxwell (1984) and Donabedian (1980). Maxwell (1984) defines quality in terms of access to services, relevance to need (for the whole community), effectiveness (for individual patients), equity (fairness), social acceptability, efficiency and economy. The Kings Fund and the Joint Committee on the Accreditation of Healthcare Organisations (JCAHO) (Ellis and Whittington, 1993) echo Maxwell's approach. Donabedian (1980) defined quality in terms of structure, process and outcome. These formulae are attempts to define the key attributes of health services in order to guide standard setting, performance measurement and review.

This raises the question: why does quality in health services need product attributes spelling out when the rest of industry gets along with *simply meeting customer requirements*? It is because health services, both in their production and their consumption, are far more complex than other kinds of industry and standard industrial quality management approaches cannot deal with this (Walsh, 1995). Each individual patient-health service episode consists of an intangible, ephemeral, unique, highly variable and contentious process that cannot just be lifted off the supermarket shelf – unlike a tin of beans (see Walsh (1998a, 1995) for a full account of the differences between an health service and a manufactured good). With the ultimate limits to medical innovation being social and moral rather than technical there will always be a 'quality gap' between what is possible and what is available (Walsh, 1995). This is the ever receding Cheshire Cat smile of health service quality. So, given the complexity of health services, how can the quality gap be filled? To understand this it is necessary to turn to Habermas (1991) to help distinguish between three kinds of quality management: *strategic*, *normative* and *critical quality*.

Strategic, Normative and Critical Quality

Jürgen Habermas, the leading contemporary thinker in the so-called Frankfurt School of *critical theory*, set out his critical social theory in a massive two volume work in the 1980s (see Habermas, 1991). This all-encompassing work is aimed at setting out the conditions under which social and technical developments, like those of health services, can serve human society without oppressing individuals or groups within it. To do this he focused on the theory of social action and undertook a massive reconstruction of contributions by theorists as diverse as Weber, Lukacs, Adorno, Mead, Durkheim, Parsons and Marx. It is broadly accepted that *action* is the conscious *human* attempt to *master a situation* (Habermas, 1990). Habermas concluded that four broad kinds of *social action* have been identified: *teleological, normatively regulated, dramaturgical* and *communicative action*. The latter is his own contribution. These represent four fundamentally different but complementary views about the way an individual can master a situation. It follows that quality management can be seen as an attempt to gain mastery over production.

Teleological (or goal-focused) action arises out of the theory that individuals are selfish goal seekers – in economic terms utility maximizers – who acquire knowledge of means in order to achieve desirable ends. Habermas applies the term *strategic* action when someone is manipulated by another as a means to an end. Even apparently cooperative behaviour in this view is nothing but utility maximizing. This far reaching assumption underpins all the recent work by public choice theorists (e.g. Dunleavy, 1991; Pirie, 1988) and health economists (Maynard, 1992; Mooney, 1991). Most famously it has given rise to Quality Adjusted Life Years (Mooney, 1991). Perhaps more significantly authors like Oakland (1993), Munroe-Faure and Munroe-Faure (1992), Hutchins (1990) and *all* the industrial 'quality gurus' also assume that quality management is aimed at improving competitiveness (in commerce) or value for money (in the NHS). In other words quality is regarded as a variable mediating between the selfish *strategic* interests of consumers and producers. I call this a condition of *strategic quality*.

Industrial examples of strategic quality are easy to find. Henry Ford famously told a customer that she could have 'any colour you like as long as its black' (Nevine, 1957, p. 188). With Ford, quality was a variable strategically specified by *one side* – the powerful producer monopolizing a market. After World War II, as Hutchins (1990) explains, Japanese producers identified specific consumer requirements of goods like cars which British producers were blind to – rust-proofing for example – leading to selective improvements advantageous to both producer and consumer. Consumers signalled their approval by buying Japanese. In other words quality came to be seen as a *two-sided* variable mediated by market forces.

Normatively regulated (rightness-focused) action is based on the view that it is natural for people to do things according to *norms*. Habermas (1991) defines a *norm* as the *entitlement* of a group of individuals to a particular (or 'right') behaviour according to circumstances. Thus *normative quality* exists when the specification of what is produced is regulated by shared expectations and entitlements. The advent of mass production and world wide distribution led to standardization in manufactured goods (Woodward, 1972) and standardization in general is one of the clearest signs of normative quality. This affects every aspect of life, from national currencies (dollar, sterling, ECUs and the proposed Euro) to three pin plugs in the UK; car exhaust emissions; screw threads; nail sizes; hygiene regulations in cafes; plumbing; building standards; University marking schemes and so on. Failing to meet standards, like those of health and safety, run the risk of sanctions which may be rule guided (you are taken to court, tribunal or you are downgraded) or market guided (no-one buys your goods).

Dramaturgical (trust-focused) action is an under – researched form that assumes that individuals can be regarded as dramatic actors. The way someone acts is assumed to be a representation of their inner-selves to others who may draw conclusions about the authenticity and sincerity of the performance. This is the basis of trust in all personal and public relationships. Politicians in an election year desperately want to be trusted. Are they speaking truthfully? Would you, as John F. Kennedy put it, buy a second hand car from this man? Will your patient believe you when you say that they need an operation? Or that nothing more can be done? Interestingly sincerity cannot be disembodied. It is judged in relation to a performance by an individual. Machines cannot be sincere. So if there is a *recorded* message of apology for a long delay played to a queue of people, will they believe it? What is there to believe? The personal touch is vital in quality management. It would be neat but it is perhaps unnecessary to define *dramaturgical quality* because the final form of social action, *communicative action*, leads to a view which accounts for this aspect of quality.

Communicative (understanding-focused) action arises out of the common sense view that people at least sometimes must communicate unreservedly in order to reach genuine understandings. This is not simply a matter of passing information on. Rather it involves willingness to discuss all the teleological (goal-focused), normative (rightness-focused) and dramaturgical (trust-focused) issues arising in a situation and offering clarification where requested. Habermas argues that this is natural and vital because the alternative strategic and normatively regulated ways to coordinate action each have serious limitations. For example, strategic action is competitive. Competition means that there are winners and losers and winning does not necessarily require any calculation of the common good. Sometimes it is better not to compete but to cooperate. On the other hand the only issue in normatively regulated action is concern as to whether *the* rule has been followed, or *the* standard has been met, not whether the rule or standard is any good. The limitations and failures of strategic and normatively regulated action can be severe, for example for people living in Northern Ireland, or for those who cannot get appropriate medical treatment for disease.

Habermas (1991) turned to *linguistics* (specifically the branch known as *universal pragmatics*) for the analysis of the assumptions implicit in communicative action. He was able to identify four specific but universal *validity claims*.

- Claims to *truth*, for example about the effectiveness of a treatment, or of the validity of a diagnostic tool.
- Claims to *rightness*, for example of a treatment or a service.
- Claims to *sincerity*, for example of a doctor's intentions, thoughts, feelings.
- The fact that language is used *at all* is a claim to *intelligibility* without which any speech or writing would be meaningless.

Although *intelligibility* is a precondition for the existence of conversation as a claim it often seems sidelined. Habermas all but ignores the issue, mainly, it seems, because 'it does not belong to pragmatics' (Holub, 1991, p. 13). However, the downplaying of intelligibility does not reflect the highly pragmatic problem of unintelligible terms cropping up constantly in conversations *especially* between clinicians and patients.

In principle all these claims can be denied or accepted by a simple *yes* or *no*. A statement of 'fact' is a claim to *truth* (such as *wounds heal more quickly with eusol*) to which the response may be *yes, I accept that what you are saying is true* or *no, I deny that what you are saying is true*. Similarly *rightness* and *sincerity* can also be accepted or denied. Of course speech is also regulated normatively and strategically. Communications can be daunting, intimidating or bureaucratically constrained, or mechanically sterilized – like recorded messages. So genuine understandings can only emerge from *dialogue* between individuals or groups under certain conditions. These are briefly:

- the willingness of participants to listen and to speak in turn;
- the ability of a participant in the discussion to deny a validity claim made by a speaker i.e. to be able to say *no*;
- the willingness of the speaker to clarify a claim to a listeners satisfaction;
- the commitment not to use force to resolve a disagreement.

The understanding that emerges is one in which participants know precisely where they have consensus, where they have dissensus and what coordinated actions they are going to take. This may include further research on matters of dissensus. The term dialogue is often used without rigour and in place of the term *negotiation* (Gregory and Walsh, 1993). Negotiation is concerned with competitive bargaining (I do this if you do that). Instead dialogue is a strict and cooperative process of moral, technical and personal argumentation which defines democracy. Democracy ceases when the use of force takes over from dialogue. For a comprehensive discussion of all these issues see Walsh (1995).

From the above it follows that *critical quality* is achieved when quality is managed through dialogue between consumers and producers (Walsh, 1995). However this implies several other conditions in addition to those of dialogue itself. Participants must have the means to change the quality of production. A dialogue that fails to try and involve everyone that is affected as well as those involved (to use Ulrich's (1993) excellent terminology) in the production and consumption of a health service is simply another example of strategic or normative quality. Since there were very few senior decision-makers involved in the Trent Quality Initiative (Gregory, Romm and Walsh, 1994) it could not achieve critical quality even though it is possible to show that dialogue did occur (Walsh, 1995).

The dialogue must be genuine. If individuals are shut out of the dialogue then for them quality is defined strategically or normatively. Making a dialogue on quality accessible may appear onerous but it does not necessarily mean that everyone has to be involved simultaneously. Rather, it means that the boundaries of the dialogue must be open to challenge and change – dialogue on membership. This is a fundamental issue. Giddens (1994) argues that political reform is needed to overturn the destruction of welfare in the 1980s and to achieve this requires that democracy should reach both up and down, from nations to individuals. Critical quality might then be seen as the main democratic element of this kind of political restructuring. Critical quality does not necessarily completely displace strategic or normatively regulated quality but it does mean that these modes of management no longer need be taken as given. So how do these concepts help with understanding the management of quality in health services?

Understanding Strategic, Normative and Critical Quality in Health Services

Florence Nightingale probably is the most famous influence on the quality of health care in the Western world. The way she improved the care of battlefield victims in the Crimean War in the mid nineteenth century is an example of strategic quality management. Using a simple scale of *relieved, unrelieved, died* to measure the outcome of care (Shaw, 1986) she demonstrated that caring practices could be improved. In doing so Nightingale displaced the existing normative quality of care and established more dynamic expectations.

At the turn of the century in Boston (USA) E.A. Codman's systematic review of medical practice involved calling back his patients after a year to check the accuracy of his diagnoses, the degree of benefits and side effects of treatment. Codman founded the 'End Results Hospital' (Ellis and Whittington, 1993). This innovation is an early example of two-sided strategic quality in health care focused upon the output of the service.

However the difficulties in undertaking anything other than very simple outcome measurements in health services has led to most developments in quality being aimed at improving the structure and process (Hutchinson, 1991). On the one hand improvements in process were confidently procured by improving the 'education and licensing of practitioners' (Ellis and Whittington, 1993, p. ll). In other words the quality of output was believed to be assured by the normative quality of medical input. For example, in the USA the Flexner Report (Flexner, 1910) on theoretical and practice standards in medical education stemmed from evaluation in medical schools commenced by the American Medical Association and the Carnegie Foundation. The Royal Colleges in the United Kingdom undertook the inspection of hospitals, departments and training programmes to check their suitability for medical student training. Other health related professional organizations followed suit. In this way normative quality of health care spread through training. Recently this has included moves to introduce regular re-licensing as a way of maintaining strategic pressure on practitioners to maintain their standards of practice (Ellis and Whittington, 1993).

The professional regulation of quality is often based upon legally enforceable entitlements by the public and the profession to work carried out according to certain explicit principles. These principles are often codified, published and put in public places such as the code of conduct for nurse, midwifes and health visitors (UKCC, 1994). The 1518 Royal Charter of the Royal College of Physicians of London is the earliest British example of a code which required that doctors uphold the standards of medicine for professional and public benefit. It is interesting to note the public centred value expressed in the code. It may have been the King's attempt at strategic quality management (it probably made him more popular) but it also formed a regal normative quality of care. The Hippocratic oath is thousands of years old but is still amongst the most well known ethical principles governing the normative quality of medical practice (Seedhouse, 1988).

On the other hand, the myriad quality initiatives in health services have been aimed at standardizing virtually everything *bar* the outcome. Ellis and Whittington identify 13 varieties of quality initiative that they classify as 'quality specific techniques' (because they were devised as means to manage quality) (1993, pp. 66–154) and 'generic techniques' (because they were devised for management generally) (ibid., pp. 155–88). They then discuss over 40 examples of quality initiative drawn from these categories that have emerged mainly in the 1980s.

It was from the 1930s onwards that outputs of care gained in importance in the UK and the USA, as a variety of studies produced useful data (ibid.). Many of these studies are continuing to the present day. They are mainly concerned with one particular kind of outcome – *death* – in a variety of settings: maternity (Hooker, 1933; Maxwell, 1984); anaesthesia (Lunn and Mushlin, 1982); and peri-operative deaths (Campling, Devlin, Hoile et al., 1993). Other outcomes of health care have been studied, such as the success of cardiac surgery, diagnostic testing and caesarian sections (Ellis and Whittington, 1993). Nevertheless, outcome studies still have been undertaken for only a minority of health services. Where high grade studies have been done they correspond somewhat to attempts at statistical process control in industry which feedback to the controller who then makes adjustments. This is complemented by an informal tradition of clinical meetings in hospitals to discuss unusual or difficult cases. Ellis and Whittington (1993) point out that this usually begins with a review of medical records which also corresponds to a methodological bias toward retrospective inspection. However, another analogy may be made: unusual or difficult medical cases are analogous to the errors that most strategic quality management methods in manufacturing seek to eliminate at source.

The Trent Quality Initiative (Gregory, Romm and Walsh, 1994) found that many staff at all levels from domestics to senior consultants were often involved in several quality initiatives, such as quality circles and standard setting for example, but that possibly only a minority of initiatives were considered to be 'working well' (Gregory et al., 1994, p. 29). This may reflect a problem that the 'efflorescence' of quality initiatives, as Ellis and Whittington (1993, p. 13) put it, may be at a very superficial level. It may also reflect a general lack of theoretical and practical insight.

All the approaches to quality dealt with by Ellis and Whittington clearly contribute to either strategic quality (by producing information of use to clinical and managerial decision makers) or normative quality (by setting standards). None of the initiatives inherently support dialogue.

Adam (1987) commented that quality in the NHS suffers from a 'partial approach'. This is echoed by Donabedian (1991) and Ellis and Whittington (1993) who argue that there is professional fragmentation of quality which is clearly visible in the way a multitude of separate records are kept for an individual patient. It is difficult to pin down who can or should be responsible for improvements or developments in quality. According to Ellis and Whittington there is a lack of 'dialogue' between the NHS professions (1993, p. 196) a view similarly expressed by Normand, Ditch, Dockrell et al. (1991) who argue that multi-disciplinary working, though supposedly widespread, is more often talked about than accomplished. Therefore the lack of critical quality in the relationship between health service producers and patients (or other external customers) is complemented by and perhaps arises out of a lack of critical quality in the relationship between health service producers (i.e. the internal customers). However for the final part of this discussion I will concentrate on critical quality in the producer-consumer relationship of the NHS.

Patient Partnership and Critical Quality

Given that producers and consumers both take part in the production of health services it is perhaps surprising how little regard has been paid to consumers by professionals. Ironically, given the consumerist ideology of the British Government of the time, Maynard (1992) commented that the role of the consumer was one of the unresolved issues of the 1989 NHS reforms. Defining this role has been on the NHS R&D agenda since at least 1991 (Peckham, 1995). James (1992, p. 5), reporting to the Department of Health on social services, stated that the 'primary definition of quality should be that of the service user'. The NHS Management Executive published a consultation document expressing the need for a 'move away from one-off consultation towards ongoing involvement of local people in purchasing activities' (National Health Service Management Executive, 1992a, p. 1). They supported the publication of research guidelines for Health Authorities to facilitate polling the views of local people about the purchase of NHS services (National Health Service Management Executive, 1992b). Walsh (1995) argues that these guidelines are aimed at providing marketing information of strategic value to purchasers (the *de facto paying* customers of the NHS (Gregory and Walsh, 1993)). In other words the guidelines only support strategic quality. So in practice the 'listening' initiative mainly resulted in limited participation in service planning and standard setting (see Gregory, Romm and Walsh, 1994) and:

> It is not surprising therefore that patient surveys and Health Service Ombudsmen reports often report concern about lack of information, poor communication and a perceived absence of real partnership in decision-making (Department of Health, 1996, p. 3, para. 7).

Clearly the level of consumer involvement has been regarded as insufficient and this led to part of the NHS Research and Development strategy being explicitly designated 'Consumers and research in the NHS' (Department of Health, 1995). From this has emerged the *Patient Partnership Strategy* (Department of Health, 1996) launched with its own senior executive (Dr Val Billingham) in 1996.

The strategy document acknowledges several influences. These are the view that planning 'on the basis of needs identified in conjunction with users' is more likely to be 'appropriate and effective'; the recognition that there is demand for openness, accountability and user 'say' on provision and standards; the view that patients want 'more information' about their care and that this is 'integral to the whole notion of informed consent'; the view that 'some evidence' indicates that user involvement improves 'health care outcomes and increases patient satisfaction'; finally the view that information about clinical effectiveness and outcomes must be communicated 'to patients in a form that they can understand' (Department of Health, 1996, p. 2, para. 4). Apparently building on these principles the strategy was divided into four overall aims:

- to promote user involvement in their own care, as active partners with professionals;

- to enable patients to become informed about their treatment and care and make informed decisions and choices about if they wish;
- to contribute to the quality of health services by making them more responsive to the needs and preferences of users;
- to ensure that users have the knowledge, skills and support to enable them to influence NHS service policy and planning.

To achieve these aims work was to be undertaken on producing and disseminating information, meeting structural, organizational and resourcing requirements (including helping users develop skills), supporting staff in partnership and undertaking further research on effective mechanisms for patient partnership and involvement (ibid., p. 5, para. 14). So will this lead to critical quality?

Steps Toward Critical Quality?

Since the launch of the patient partnership strategy there have been a large number of local NHS patient partnership initiatives (Department of Health, 1997a, b). Many have the potential to contribute to critical quality. For example the Phoenix NHS Trust has service user forums and have been designing a policy for learning disabled user involvement in staff appointments (Phoenix NHS Trust, 1997). 'Citizens juries' are currently seen as a fashionable possibility for tackling local health service decisions (Kings Fund, 1997). However many initiatives appear aimed more simply at enabling NHS professionals to 'milk' information and opinions from NHS users (e.g. Taylor, Dunlop and Stevenson, 1997). What use is made of this data is up to the professionals. This, like most current initiatives, may lead to some strategic changes in quality and eventually a new normative quality of health service – but not to critical quality. Another possibility raised during the Trent Quality Initiative is that Community Health Councils might provide an advocacy service to help patients clarify what aspects of clinical decisions they want to challenge, with a view to reaching an understanding with clinicians. Some advocacy schemes are in progress (e.g. Kurtiz, Pownceby and Cowperthwaite, 1997). Few, if any, initiatives seem focused on the problem of informed consent, perhaps because there is a feeling that this 'problem' is intractable. Why is this?

Informed Consent and Clinical Decision-making

Informed consent is a keystone in the patient partnership strategy. The strategy view is that more and better information packaged appropriately is needed to enable actively involved patients to make informed choices. Yet this implies a serious misconception about the nature of informed consent. The main problem with informed consent is not *lack of information*. Rather it is *lack of understanding*. This is caused by the lack of a suitable process through which patients can reach understandings with clinicians. All clinical decisions need evidence in the form of facts, experiences and information to support claims of intelligibility, truth, rightness and sincerity each of which can lead to a demand by patients for clarification. All these demands have to be met to the satisfaction of the patient. Otherwise there can be no understanding and *no informed consent* (Walsh, 1998a). Indeed the idea that more and better measurements of diseases, treatments, attitudes, satisfaction, *etc. necessarily* must lead to better quality is wrong. More and better technical knowledge is useless from a lay or patient's perspective unless it is fed into a process of dialogue in which patients can reach an understanding with the clinician. It also follows that no clinical course of action can be justified on an expert view of effectiveness or outcome criteria alone no matter how well supported scientifically. All the claims have equal weight – if one is not fulfilled then there is a serious flaw in the rationality of the decision. Such weaknesses may lead to questions being asked later about the competence, intentions or moral rectitude of the clinician. What is needed to establish critical quality in clinical decision making is a competent process through which clinical evidence (in the form of facts, experiences and information) is discussed openly by those who are affected by the decision *with the purpose of reaching mutual understanding*.

This does not mean that patients have to know as much as clinicians in order to say *yes* or *no* to validity claims. It simply means recognizing that *patients* decide whether the evidence is good enough *for them*. This is 'a matter of judgment and an exercise in practical wisdom' (Walsh, 1991, p. 505). For example a patient may not know the ins and outs of heart surgery but they may want to know how their surgeon's mortality rate compares with her or his peers. In response the surgeon may be able to demonstrate that her/his mortality rate is insignificant compared to other causes of mortality, and so on. The main barrier to dialogue is not the complexity of the issue or the patients lack of scientific knowledge. Instead it is the lack of time for and commitment to *an adequate process of dialogue*. The strategy currently does not refer to dialogue and will not, as it stands, lead to critical quality in clinical decision-making or anything other than a re-mix of the current strategic/normative quality balance of the NHS. This will never be regarded as satisfactory and unattenuated public expectations will probably continue to be exploited politically and socially. Everyone should expect the NHS to be reformed again in vain attempts to close the quality gap. There is considerable demand for genuine public involvement in NHS decision making. Hence the only reform that will last is one in which dialogue processes are implemented in clinical, local and national decision making. In other words, reforms that are aimed at the comprehensive achievement of critical quality. Gregory, Romm and Walsh (1994) provide one design for dialogue at a local multi-agency level of health service decision making. Urgent research is necessary on the design of dialogue on clinical and national health service decision-making.

References

Adam, C. (1987), 'Creating a Quality Service' in Department of Community Medicine (eds), *Creating Quality in the NHS, Occasional Papers No. 11*, University of Manchester, Manchester.

Campling, E. A., Devlin, H.B., Hoile, R. W. et al. (1993), *The Report of the National Confidential Enquiry into Peri-operative Deaths 1991/2*, National Confidential Enquiry into Peri-operative Deaths, London.

Crosby, P.B. (1979), *Quality is Free*, Mentor, New York.

Deming, W.E. (1982), *Out of the Crisis*, MIT, Cambridge, Massachusetts.

Department of Health (1995), *Consumers and Research in the NHS: An R&D contribution to consumer involvement in the NHS*, Department of Health, Leeds.

Department of Health (1996), *Patient Partnership Strategy*, Department of Health, Leeds.

Donabedian, A. (1980), *The Definition of Quality and Approaches to its Assessment*, Ann Arbor, Michigan.

Donabedian, A. (1991), 'Reflections on the Effectiveness of Quality Assurance' in R.H. Palmer (ed.), *Striving for Quality in Health Care*, Ann Arbor, Michigan.

Dunleavy, P. (1991), *Democracy, Bureaucracy and Public Choice*, Harvester Wheatsheaf, London.

Ellis, R. and Whittington, D. (1993), *Quality Assurance in Health Care*, Edward Arnold, London.

Flexner, A. (1910), *Medical Education in the United States and Canada*, Carnegie Foundation, New York.

Giddens, A. (1994), 'Agenda Change', *New Society and Statesmen*, 7 October, pp. 23–5.

Gregory, W., Romm, N.R.A. and Walsh, M.P. (1994), 'The Trent Quality Initiative: A multi-agency evaluation of quality standards in the National Health Service', research report, Centre for Systems Studies, University of Hull.

Gregory, W. and Walsh, M. (1993), *Quality, Ideology and Consumer Choice* in M. Malek, P. Vacani and J. Rasquinhi (eds), Managerial Issues in the reformed NHS, John Wiley, Chichester.

Habermas, J. (1990), *Moral Consciousness and Communicative Action*, Polity, Cambridge.

Habermas, J. (1991), *The Theory of Communicative Action*, Vol. 1, Polity, Cambridge.

Holub, R.C. (1991), *Jürgen Habermas: Critic in the Public Sphere*, Routledge, London.

Hooker, R.S. (1933), *Maternity Mortality in New York City: A study of all puerperal deaths*, Oxford University Press, New York.

Hutchins, D. (1990), *In Pursuit of Quality*, Pitman, London.

Hutchinson, A. (1991), Inaugural Lecture, Department of Public Health Medicine, University of Hull.

Ishikawa, K. and Lu, D.J. (1985), *What is Total Quality Control?*, Prentice Hall, Englewood Cliffs, New Jersey.

James, A. (1992), *Committed to Quality: Quality assurance in social services departments*, HMSO, London.

Juran, J.M. (1988), *Quality Control Handbook*, McGraw Hill, New York.

Kings Fund (1997), 'Citizens' Juries', presented at Department of Health conference *Patient Partnership – what's in it for me?*, 21 May, Queen Elizabeth Conference Centre, London.

Kurtiz, J., Pownceby, J. and Cowperthwaite, C. (1997), 'Patient Advocacy in a Cystic Fibrosis Centre', presented at Department of Health conference *Patient Partnership – what's in it for me?*, 21 May, Queen Elizabeth Conference Centre, London.

Lunn, J.N. and Mushlin, W.W. (1982), *Mortality Associated with Anaesthesia*, Nuffield Provincial Hospitals Trust, London.

Maxwell, R. (1984), 'Quality assessment in health', *British Medical Journal*, 289, pp. 1470–2.

Maynard, A. (1992), *Competition in Health Care: Whatever happened to the government health reforms?*, Smith and Nephew Lecture, Department of Social Policy and Professional Studies, University of Hull, Hull.

Mooney, G. (1991), *Economics, Medicine and Health Care*, Harvester Wheatsheaf, London.

Munroe-Faure, L. and Munroe-Faure, M. (1992), *Total Quality Management*, Pitman, London.

National Health Service Management Executive (1992a), *Local Voices: The views of local people in purchasing for health, January 1992*, Department of Health, Leeds.

National Health Service Management Executive (1992b), *Listening to Local Voices*, Department of Health, Leeds.

Nevine, A. (1957), *Oxford Book of Quotations*, Oxford University Press, Oxford.

Normand, C., Ditch, J., Dockerell, J. et al. (1991), *Clinical Audit in the Professions Allied to Medicine*, Health and Health Care Research Unit, Belfast.

Oakland, J.S. (1993), *Total Quality Management: The route to improving performance*, Butterworth-Heinemann, Oxford.

Peckham, M. (1995), 'Consumers and Research in the NHS: Foreword' in *Consumers and Research in the NHS: An R&D contribution to consumer involvement in the NHS*, Department of Health, Leeds.

Phoenix NHS Trust (1997), *Information sheet on Patient Partnership Initiatives*, Phoenix NHS Trust, Stoke Park, Stapleton, Bristol, BS16 1QU.

Pirie, M. (1988), *Micropolitics*, Wildwood House, London.

Seedhouse, D. (1988), *Ethics – the heart of healthcare*, John Wiley, Chichester.

Shaw, C. (1986), *Quality Assurance: What the Royal Colleges are doing*, King Edwards Hospital Fund, London.

Taylor, A., Dunlop, P. and Stevenson, P. (1997), 'Teeside Talks Back', presented at Department of Health conference *Patient Partnership – what's in it for me?*, 21 May, Queen Elizabeth Conference Centre, London.

UKCC (1994), *Code of Conduct for Nurses, Mid-wifes, and Health Visitors*, United Kingdom Central Council for Nursing, London.

Ulrich, W. (1994), *Critical Heuristics of Social Planning: A new approach to practical philosophy*, John Wiley & Sons, Chichester.

Walsh, K. (1991), 'Quality and public services', *Public Administration*, 69 (winter), pp. 503–14.

Walsh, M.P. (1995), 'Critical Systems Thinking, Dialogue and Quality Management in the National Health Service', PhD thesis, University of Hull.

Walsh, M.P. (1998a), 'What is evidence? a critical view for nursing', *Journal of Clinical Effectiveness in Nursing*, forthcoming.

Walsh, M.P. (1998b), 'Beyond TQM in health services', paper for the *Third International Conference on Strategic Issues in Health Care Management*, 2–4 April, University of St Andrews.

Woodward, C.D. (1972), *British Standards Institute: The story of standards*, British Standards Institute, Milton Keynes.

4 Whose Quality? Different Interest Groups' Perspectives on Health Care Quality

JUAN I. BAEZA AND MICHAEL CALNAN

Centre for Health Services Studies, University of Kent

Background

It has become conventional wisdom for the evaluation of quality of health care to be divided up in to structure, process and outcome (Donobedian, 1980). This is a systems approach to the analysis of quality that appears to imply that there is agreement over how quality is defined by the major parties involved in the provision and use of health care. However, other writers have suggested that managers, clients and professionals might have differing and even conflicting perspectives about health service quality (Ovretveit, 1992): according to Grol et al. (1993), these three groups have differing priorities and place importance on different components. For example, a manager's quality goal of cost containment may clash with a professional's perspective of providing the best treatment possible. A number of authors, for example Best (1983) commenting on NHS performance indicators and Ranade (1994) on the Patient's Charter, have made similar observations that the pursuit of one quality standard may impinge on the quest for another. However, the resultant standards which are in place and acted upon will depend on which of these different interest groups are most influential (Williamson, 1992). It has been suggested (Ranade, 1994) that despite the emergence of the so-called 'new managerialism', concepts of quality in health care are still determined largely by health professionals.

This issue of the different interest groups' perspectives on quality was explored in a study evaluating the quality standards set by a general practice

Managing Quality: Strategic Issues in Health Care Management, H.T.O. Davies, M. Tavakoli, M. Malek, A.R. Neilson (eds), Ashgate Publishing Ltd, 1999.

multifund in their contracts for outpatient services. This has been a neglected area (Flynn et al., 1996) for research and this study specifically examined how quality standards were derived, adopted and what impact they had, the acceptability and importance of the standards, and more broadly how quality was defined. Each of these questions was explored from the point of view of the different interest groups.

The research presented here focuses on one case study of a large multifund situated in the southeast of England (see Baeza and Calnan, 1997a). The focus of the research was organized around the contracting process and more specifically on quality standards in the multifund's contracts for outpatient services with its main provider.

The methodology adopted both qualitative and quantitative techniques. Data on the derivation and impact of the quality standards, along with broader views about quality, were elicited through face-to-face tape-recorded interviews with key actors in the contracting process. This involved two rounds of interviews with doctors and managers from the purchaser and provider sides. The first round consisted of 24 interviews conducted between November 1995 and May 1996 and the second round consisted of interviews with the same informants where this was possible (N = 18) which were carried out between March and June 1997. The first interviews focused specifically on the formulation and adoption of the quality standards and the second round on their impact, but also informants' views on what quality meant to them in general and the most appropriate way of enhancing quality.

The quantitative element consisted of surveys of a random sample of recent users of the outpatient services and of the population of health care professionals involved directly or indirectly with the provision of outpatient services. The user survey finished with an achieved sample of 354 that represented a 58 per cent response rate. The postal questionnaire investigated users' views about their awareness, acceptability and importance of the quality standards used by the multifund in its outpatient contract, as well as levels of satisfaction with their experience of their last outpatient visit. The questionnaire mailed to health professionals (consultants, hospital nurses, hospital managers, GPs, practice nurses and fundholding managers) focused on their awareness, acceptability and importance of the quality standards adopted in the contract for outpatient services. The achieved sample was 127, representing an overall response rate of 60 per cent.

The Construction of Quality Standards

What follows is a summary of the data (for a fuller version, see Baeza and Calnan, 1997b). There was a general consensus from GPs, consultants and health service managers on the importance of having standards mainly, because they provided targets to aim for. However, the managers, not surprisingly, saw it as a way of monitoring performance, for example, as a hospital manager stated:

> ... you have a standard there and you either achieve that standard or you can't achieve that standard, if you can partly achieve that then you have the opportunity of totally achieving it in the future if you make changes or whatever. If you don't have written standards you have no way of measuring.

The major feature of the way the standards were constructed was that it was perceived by the informants as being non-participatory. This might reflect a lack of interest in the quality standards, particularly by the health professionals from both the purchasing and provider side. From the GPs' point of view the quality standards were seen as an issue for management to deal with, which was the very reason for their joining the multifund in the first place, in that they were keen to escape managerial obligations (Audit Commission, 1996). For example, as one multifund GP representative stated:

> Well, I won't say they're not interested, they certainly don't know, I'm sure my partners haven't a clue about what the quality standards in the contracts are. [...] Most GPs are not terribly interested in the mechanics, they just want to get their patients in and get a good opinion.

Similarly there was a lack of interest and concern over the quality standards from the hospital consultants, particularly as there are no penalties or incentives for adhering to them. This is how one consultant saw it:

> ... I have to say we don't achieve all the quality standards. Well again you see the problem is there's ... no real penalty at the end of the day when you haven't achieved it and if there was I guess we'd be in there fighting much more at the beginning because that's what it should be.

Furthermore, our research would suggest that, due to a lack of monitoring and evaluation of the quality standards, on many occasions the multifund would be unaware whether the standards are being met or not.

Professional, Managerial and User Acceptability

The aim of presenting data from the two surveys of users, health professionals and managerial views on the awareness, acceptability and importance of the quality standards was to shed light on how the groups' perspectives might be similar or different with regard to quality.

The evidence from the surveys suggests that the user–professional–manager distinction might be simplistic. The acceptability of many of the multifund's standards was high across all the three categories. Where there were marked variations in perspectives it was usually between hospital doctors and general practitioners, and additionally there were differences between those on the purchasing and providing side. These differences are illustrated by Figures 4.1 and 4.2, which asked the various groups' acceptability of two quality standards that are contained in the multifund's outpatient contracts.

A routine outpatient appointment will be available within 12 weeks with at least one consultant in any specialty with the exception of 10 specialties

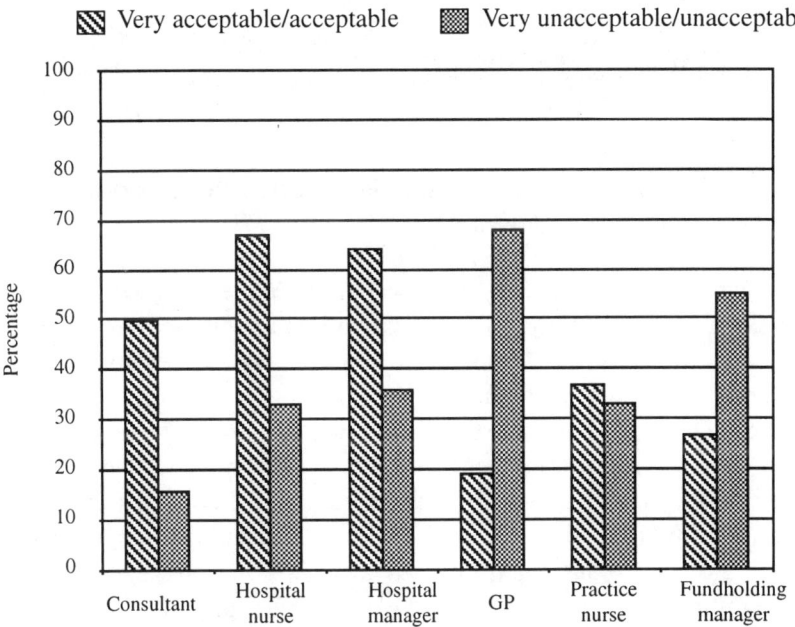

Figure 4.1 The acceptability of a standard on waiting times for an outpatient appointment

The number of follow-ups following an operation is to be a maximum of two, except for cancers. The outpatient doctor will inform the GP when a further appointment is necessary. Lack of comment can be taken as consent for a further appointment

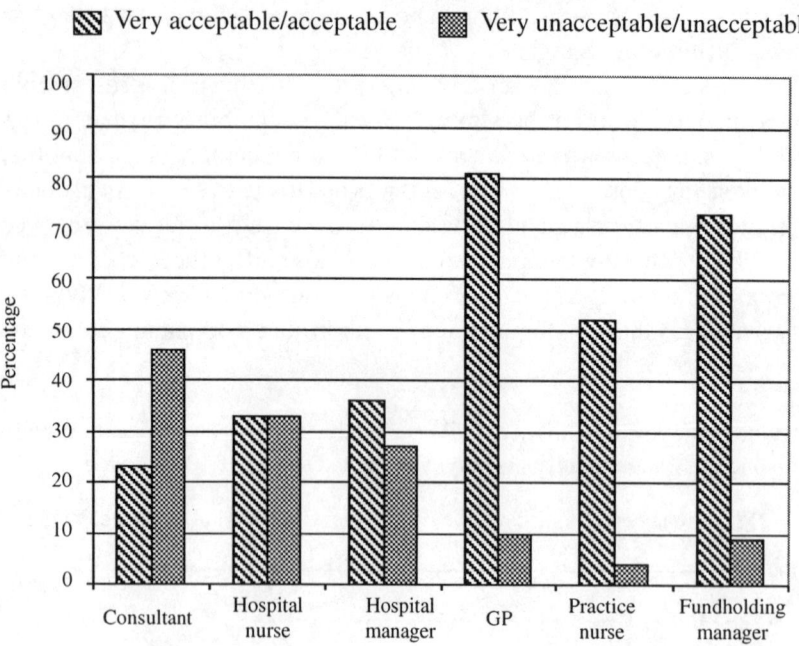

Figure 4.2   The acceptability of a standard stating the maximum number of follow-ups

It is clear from the two graphs above that there is quite a marked dichotomy in terms of the acceptability of these two particular standards between the health care professionals from the provider trust (represented by the consultants, hospital nurses and hospital managers) and those from the purchaser side (represented by the GPs, practice nurses and fundholding managers). Within these differences, however, the graphs show that it was the GPs from the purchaser side who displayed the highest levels of unacceptability and acceptability respectively of these two standards. It is also interesting to note in Figure 4.2 that hospital consultants show the highest degree of unacceptability towards a standard which could impinge on their clinical freedom, while their hospital colleagues (hospital nurses and hospital managers) are less concerned about this standard. Nevertheless, there was little evidence of any wide differences in perspective between the managers and health care professionals; the differences were, instead, between purchasers and providers, that is to say the differences were intraprofessional rather than interprofessional.

The differences were particularly evident between hospital consultants and GPs, illustrated by the answers given to the open-ended questions asked in the survey. In answer to a question asking which issues quality standards should cover, over a third of the hospital consultants who answered stated that the quality of care given in the outpatient department should be addressed, issues such as clinical effectiveness and outcomes were mentioned. On the other hand, only four of the GPs who answered mentioned these issues; their main concern was the length of waiting times for their patients' outpatient appointments. Respondents from the provider side mentioned that quality standards had resource implications. Lastly, nearly a quarter of the consultants who responded stated that quality standards should be set for the referrals that GPs make to the outpatient department.

Similarly, hospital doctors and users were in disagreement or, put another way, users had more in common with general practitioners. This was well illustrated in relation to the general issue of waiting times. The only two standards that registered any notable level of unacceptability amongst the users were concerned with waiting times. The satisfaction rates of the outpatient services amongst those users who responded were also very high. The lowest satisfaction rates were recorded for the waiting times between seeing their GP and their outpatient attendance and the amount of time they had to wait in the outpatient department before their consultation. Nearly a fifth of respondents felt these were either very unacceptable or unacceptable. It is important to note that the issue of waiting times produced the highest rates of dissatisfaction amongst users, which is the same issue that GPs considered as important in their survey.

Health Care Quality

The semi-structured interviews were used to examine the various informants' perspectives of quality. The informants were asked what they considered to be a good quality health care service. Everyone agreed that delivering a high quality service was important: however, there were differences in emphasis amongst the different health care professionals and all the informants recognized the financial constraints on the service. Informants recognized that the measurement of quality was difficult and multifaceted; it was not something that could be easily defined. A non-fundholding GP argued that:

> ... the measurement of quality in general practice is almost certainly doomed to
> failure because there are so many different parameters by which you can measure
> quality [...] I think it is almost impossible to measure the quality of an individual
> in general practice [...] So really when you ask, 'how do you measure quality
> in general practice?' I suppose my answer is 'pass'.

Although the informants found it difficult to define a good quality service,
it was recognized that there was a growing emphasis within the NHS on
delivering good quality health care. The multifund medical manager
commented:

> I think there's far more emphasis on it now. I mean, when I went into general
> practice basically GPs did what GPs do, full stop, end of story. Now, the catch
> phrases of 'clinical effectiveness', 'evidence based healthcare' are very much
> to the fore and I think that when you've been a GP for a while a lot of us feel
> that what we want to know is what we're doing valuable or not?

However, GPs had a clearer idea of what they considered a good quality
hospital service, prompt and accurate consultations were sought from their
hospital colleagues. As one GP stated:

> Well I suppose it's one that answers questions you've asked and does it quite
> quickly and who doesn't keep on seeing them endlessly for no particular benefit.

The issue of outpatient waiting times was again the most frequent issue
mentioned in the interviews by the GPs. The following GP expressed a very
common view amongst the GPs interviewed:

> We have clinical meetings when we discuss a lot of clinical problems. One of
> our constant problems is obviously patients being seen in a reasonable period
> of time. [...] The most important thing when you're sitting with a patient is to
> try to assess if they need a hospital service, and it's only a very small proportion
> of the people we're seeing who do, they need it in a reasonable space of time
> and that's the constant aggravation of our general practice.

On the other hand, the hospital consultants argued that trying to keep
waiting lists for outpatient appointments down without extra resources could
have a negative impact on quality, demonstrating that the pursuit of one quality
goal can often clash with another:

... the trouble is then if you say right, well, actually we're not going to get more resources but you still have to keep within those parameters then you tend to see more people quicker so that can affect your quality standards and if you're trying to stay within the same clinic time and you've seen more people to keep your waiting list down then that clearly could compromise quality.

The hospital consultants also found it difficult to articulate what they defined as good quality health care. Components such as audit, good outcomes and professionalism were considered important as the following comments made by hospital consultants illustrate:

... an academic input and output and time made aside for appropriate audit and research is an essential ingredient.

Well, I think the major guiding force really is one's professionalism. One wants to deliver a service as high in quality as possible. So if there are any better ways of doing things than you've been used to then one should, one's professionalism really dictates that you should be adopting the new techniques.

I suppose a good quality service would be achieved when you have a good clinical outcome as far as whatever medical condition the patient had with a satisfied patient at the end of it. Perhaps one has to add these days delivered in a relatively cost effective way.

The outpatient manager who had a long work history in the private sector had a more tangible view of what a good quality service was:

Immediately I would look at the environment. If the environment was clean and cosy I suppose. [...] The receptionists and the people that the patients meet should be polite, courteous and give answers, immediate answers rather than vague ones.

The issue of finance was often mentioned in relation to quality. Many informants felt that a good quality service depended to a certain extent on having an appropriate level of resources. A senior nurse in the outpatient department expressed this widespread belief:

I think perhaps there's a danger, as the financial restrictions are so hard now, that quality is going to start falling by the wayside because quality does cost I think. Not all of it but if you want to get new ideas going you do need some resources there and I think there are going to be a lot of potentially good ideas going down the pan.

The growing number of outreach clinics is a good example of how the various professionals have different views on what represents a good quality service. These clinics were frequently mentioned by GPs as characterizing a good quality service for patients. The following comment by a multifund GP illustrates this view:

> I mean certainly it's an improvement that patients can get more seen locally. That is a distinct improvement. Whether these out-reach clinics are good from an organizational point of view I don't know. They're very good for patients. Patients like them rather than travelling all the way up to [their local hospital].

However, one multifund GP had reservations about out-reach clinics: she felt they were restrictive and doubted their cost-effectiveness.

> I have great reservations because I feel that, first of all it limits who you refer people to. Actually if you had a surgeon coming down to do a clinic between 6.00 and 7.00 once a week you are actually going to be limited to referring all your surgical cases to him and there is specialization within surgery so I think that's better really. […] And I also feel that at the end of the day you're actually paying someone twice for doing the same job, which I think morally, I'm very against.

It was recognized by most of the informants who mentioned the issue of out-reach clinics that there were two sides to the issue which are important to appreciate. The multifund manager stated the advantages, as she saw them, of in-house clinics:

> It depends on your point of view but some would argue that they should be in the hospital, others will argue that it's perfectly reasonable. They see so many more patients because they're in a different set-up. The patients are pleased to be there in a GP's surgery where they feel their doctor has given them the appointment to be seen at their own surgery. People don't DNA or if they can't make an appointment they ring and say, so that's given to somebody else, so you get very little wastage. And it's cheaper, because you've not got all the hospital overheads and things.

The consultants who were interviewed were dubious about the benefits of the clinics. They felt that on the whole it was generally an inappropriate service to offer when there was so much sub-specialization in modern medicine. The following consultant also stated what he thought the incentives for such services might be:

Now we're getting into the realms of sub-specialization in general surgery in a very big and very rapid manner and the GPs have got to understand this process and that is one of the reasons where individual consultants popping off to do out-reach clinics is in my judgement beginning to be counterproductive. It's a convenience for the GPs because it's cheap. It's a convenience for the patients because it's local. It's a bonus for the consultants because they get backhanders, but actually whether that's the right way of doing it I really don't know. [...] You come and do an outreach clinic in my surgery which gives me good kudos with my patients and you can have all my private practice.

This same consultant gave a concrete example of what he saw as the disadvantages of such arrangements:

I saw a lady who'd been waiting for a month to see me with a breast lump because that was the next time I was going to be there whereas we'd have seen her within two days at the hospital if she'd come up to the referral practice. So there is a down side.

Discussion

The aim of this chapter was to examine the way the different interest groups conceptualize and define quality of care, drawing on a case study evaluating quality standards in the provision of hospital outpatient services. Our particular interest was how the groups differed in perspectives and whether it was possible to differentiate these perspectives according to whether they managed, provided, purchased or used the service.

The evidence from the study showed that this analytical distinction was simplistic and what divided perspectives was the setting in which care was provided, i.e. general practice compared with the hospital, and which side of the internal market they were working in. Clearly, the proposition that GPs should be advocates for their patients' interests has some support from this evidence, as GPs seemed to be more aware of patients' perspectives than their colleagues in the hospital. The hospital consultants put more emphasis on the clinical outcome of care, whereas general practitioners shared users' views about processial aspects such as waiting times and outreach clinics that are more accessible to patients.

With regard to the difference between the purchaser–provider perspective on quality, it appeared that GPs and fundholding managers put emphasis on performance and processial activities whereas their counterparts on the provider side put their emphasis on outcomes. It appears, therefore, that the provider–purchaser split might have exacerbated the differences between the GP and the hospital consultant.

Evidence suggests that the development of effective standards for quality requires participation and cooperation between all the different interest groups (North of England Study of Standards and Performance in General Practice, 1992; Onion et al., 1996; Grol, 1990). The internal market has seemed to act as a further impediment to the development of this collaboration between professionals and managers in the two different settings. The recent White Paper (*The New NHS*, 1997), which proposes to dismantle the contracting process in favour of commissioning, may go some way to fostering collaboration. In terms of quality as a whole, while most of the informants adhered to its importance, many still found it a difficult concept to define and operationalize.[1]

Note

1   The study that this chapter is based on was funded by the South Thames NHS Executive Research and Development Project Grant Scheme.

References

Audit Commission (1996), *What the Doctor Ordered: A study of GP fundholders in England and Wales*, HMSO, London.

Baeza, J.I. and Calnan, M. (1997a), 'Implementing Quality: a study of the adoption and implementation of quality standards in the contracting process in a general practitioner multifund', *Journal of Health Services Research and Policy*, 4, pp. 205–11.

Baeza, J.I. and Calnan, M. (1997b), *Evaluation of Quality Standards used by General Practitioner Fundholders in Setting Contracts*, Centre for Health Services Studies, University of Kent.

Best, G. (1983), 'Performance indicators: a precautionary tale for unit managers' in I. Wickings (ed.), *Effective Unit Management*, Kings Fund, London.

Department of Health (1997), *The New NHS*, HMSO, London.

Donabedian, A. (1982), *The Criteria and Standards of Quality: Explorations in quality, assessment and monitoring, Vol. II*, Health Administration Press, Michigan.

Flynn, R., Williams, G. and Pickard, S. (1996), *Markets and Networks: Contracting in Community Health Services*, Open University Press, Buckingham.

Grol, R. (1990), 'National standard setting for quality of care in general practice: attitudes of general practitioners and response to a set of standards', *British Journal of General Practice*, 40, pp. 361–4.

Grol, R., Wensing, M., Jacobs, A. and Baker, R. (eds) (1993), *Quality Assurance in General Practice: The state of the art in Europe*, Nederlands Huisartsen Genootschap, Utrecht.

North of England Study of Standards and performance in General Practice (1992), 'Medical Audit in General Practice', *British Medical Journal*, 304, pp. 1480–4.

Onion, C., Dutton, T., Walley, T., Turnbull, C., Dunne, W. and Buchan, I. (1996), 'Local clinical guidelines: description and evaluation of a participative method for their development and implementation', *Family Practice*, 13, pp. 28–34.

Ovretveit, J. (1992), *Health Service Quality*, Blackwell Scientific Press, Oxford.

Ranade, W. (1994), *A Future for the NHS? Health Care in the 1990s*, Longman, London.

Williamson, C. (1992), *Whose Standards? Consumer and professional standards in health care*, Open University Press, Buckingham.

5   The Quantification of Patient Satisfaction

MIKE HART
King Alfred's University College, Winchester

Introduction

Whilst the tradition of 'listening to the patients' is almost as long as the NHS itself, the prominence given to the patient satisfaction survey can be traced back to the Griffiths Report (DHSS, 1983) which encouraged the use of market research to obtain consumers' views. Purchasing authorities have been urged to pay more heed to locally expressed views of the quality of the service since the early 1990s (NHSME, 1992). It has also been recognized for about the same length of time that in judging the quality of hospital services, the judgments of patients alongside their clinicians is an intrinsic part of the quality measurement process (Batalden and Nelson, 1990).

Patient satisfaction surveys are often seen as the natural outcome of the increase in consumerism, particularly as stimulated by Griffiths. However, several authors point out that patient satisfaction surveys are used to fulfil other multiple objectives, including Quality Audit (QA) of the quality of medical and nursing care on the one hand, and the derivation of an outcome measure for the evaluation of care and the organization of services on the other (Scott and Smith, 1994; Avis, Bond and Arthur, 1995).

Dissatisfaction with the Conduct of the Patient Satisfaction Survey

There is some concern, expressed cogently by Carr-Hill (1992) after his review of some 300 patient satisfaction surveys, that the majority of them are producer-led.

Managing Quality: Strategic Issues in Health Care Management, H.T.O. Davies, M. Tavakoli, M. Malek, A.R. Neilson (eds), Ashgate Publishing Ltd, 1999.

Once the fieldwork is over, there is considerable temptation to forget that what are confidently described as respondents' views are only their replies to questions devised by the researcher and not necessarily the patients' own views and priorities. Thus it is commonplace to observe that health service policy has been steered by providers' perceptions and definitions of good practice (Carr-Hill, 1992, p. 245).

Carr-Hill is also concerned with the many methodological inadequacies which he details as a result of his survey. These range from problems with the framing of the questions, the avoidance of evaluation of clinical practice, the inadequate ways in which samples relate to the populations from which they are drawn and the cavalier treatment of non-response rates. To this, we may add the fact that many patient surveys appear to exhibit a halo effect, in which satisfaction rates seem to be uniformly high at over 80 per cent, perhaps reflecting a reluctance to criticize nurses (Carr-Hill, 1992; Fitzpatrick, 1991a, 1991b; Evason and Whittington, 1991; Ellis and Whittington, 1994; College of Health, 1994). There are indications, however, that much more attention is now being paid to questionnaires in terms of both their construct validity (Baker and Whitfield, 1992) and their reliability/validity (Bamford and Jacoby, 1992; Eccles, Jacoby and Bamford, 1992). The timing and location of the survey may itself be a critical factor. In a study of particular relevance to a concern with outpatients (Carr-Hill, Humphreys and McIver, 1987), it is shown that there is a clear decay in satisfaction levels when patients are interviewed at home rather than in the outpatient clinic. But probably the greatest single source of dissatisfaction with the traditional survey is its superficiality. The most common method of data collection involves the use of pre-coded self-completion questionnaires (Batchelor, Owens, Read and Bloor, 1994; Scott and Smith, 1994). But as Rigge (1995, pp. 26–7) has pointed out:

> Handing out tick-in-the-box patient satisfaction questionnaires and then sitting smugly back if the results indicate that most patients are satisfied with the service they have received (as many such quantitative methods do) is no substitute for genuine consultation.

Measurement of Service Quality – the SERVQUAL Methodology

Unlike the quality of goods, which can be measured objectively by such indicators as durability and number of defects, service quality is an abstract and elusive construct because of three features unique to services: intangibility, heterogeneity and inseparability of production and consumption.

The SERVQUAL methodology is primarily developed to measure satisfaction with service industries. The method is well-known in total quality management circles. The approach starts with the hypothesis that service quality is critically determined by the difference between consumers' expectations and perceptions of services. The method is predicated upon the gap to be discerned between clients' expectations of a service and their perceptions of a service as actually experienced.

Research by Parasuraman, Zeithaml and Berry (1988) has shown that regardless of the type of service, consumers use basically similar criteria in evaluating service quality. The criteria fall into 10 key categories which are labelled 'service quality determinants' as follows:

1 *reliability*, which involves consistency of performance and dependability;

2 *responsiveness* concerns the willingness or readiness of employees to provide service. It involves timeliness of service;

3 *competence* means possession of the required skills and knowledge to perform the service;

4 *access* involves approachability and ease of contact;

5 *courtesy* involves politeness, respect, consideration and friendliness of contact personnel;

6 *communication* means keeping customers informed in language they can understand and listening to them;

7 *credibility* involves trustworthiness, believability and honesty. It involves having the customer's best interests at heart;

8 *security* is the freedom from danger, risk or doubt;

9 *understanding/knowing the customer* involves making the effort to understand the customer's needs;

10 *tangibles* include the physical evidence of the service like physical facilities and appearance of personnel.

Only two of the 10 determinants – tangibles and credibility – can be known in advance of delivery, the others often only being evidenced once a service transaction has taken place. While customers may possess some information based on their experience or on other customers' evaluations, they are likely to re-evaluate these determinants each time a service is given because of the heterogeneity of services. Consumers cannot evaluate two of the determinants – competence and security – even after service delivery and consumption.

The gap between expectations and perceptions may be analysed with respect to five dimensions. An examination of the content of the 10 service quality items allows a construction of five dimensions in SERVQUAL, of which three are original list items (*tangibles, reliability, responsiveness*) and two are combined dimensions: (*assurance*, including communication, credibility, security, competence and courtesy; *empathy*, including understanding/knowing customers and access). The final list of five dimensions and their concise definitions is as follows:

1 *tangibles*: physical facilities, equipment and appearance of personnel;

2 *reliability*: ability to perform the promised service dependably and accurately;

3 *responsiveness*: willingness to help customers and provide prompt service;

4 *assurance*: knowledge and courtesy of employees and their ability to inspire trust and confidence;

5 *empathy*: caring, individualized attention the firm provides its customers.

The last two dimensions contain items representing seven original dimensions (communication, credibility, security, competence, courtesy, understanding/knowing customers and access) that did not remain distinct after the two stages of scale purification. Therefore, while SERVQUAL has only five distinct dimensions, they capture facets of all 10 originally conceptualized dimensions.

In the questionnaires the dimensions are divided into a 22 item, seven point scale. Dimensions may not be regarded as equally important. Each client may allocate points out of 100 to each of the five dimensions so that the instrument is sensitive to an individual's perceptions of the relative importance of each dimension.

SERVQUAL has a variety of potential applications. It can help a wide range of service and retailing organizations in assessing consumer expectations about and perceptions of service quality. It can also help in pinpointing areas requiring managerial attention and action to improve service quality.

Application of SERVQUAL can be used to make comparisons globally over time. Moreover, it is possible to ascertain those elements of services in which the gap between expectations and perceptions is widest. The application of this instrument and the results of measurement allows possibilities of more specific management action to redress perceived shortcomings. Although well-developed and extensively used in USA, studies are only just commencing utilising the methodology within the UK and Finland (Tables 5.1–5.3).

Table 5.1   SERVQUAL results – previous studies: USA general sample (1990)

Dimension	Weight	Perceptions	Expectations	Gap
Tangibles	0.11	5.54	5.16	+0.38
Reliability	0.32	5.16	6.44	-1.28
Responsiveness	0.22	5.20	6.36	-1.16
Assurance	0.19	5.50	6.50	-1.00
Empathy	0.16	5.16	6.28	-1.12
Weighted averages (n = 1,936)		5.28	6.27	-0.99

Source: calculated from Zeithaml, Parasuraman and Berry, 1990.

Table 5.2   East Midlands, UK outpatients (July 1995)

Dimension	Weight	Perceptions	Expectations	Gap
Tangibles	0.13	5.21	5.24	-0.03
Reliability	0.26	5.52	6.31	-0.79
Responsiveness	0.21	5.88	6.17	-0.29
Assurance	0.20	5.98	6.39	-0.41
Empathy	0.20	5.66	6.16	-0.50
Weighted averages (n = 72)		5.67	6.15	-0.48

Table 5.3   Vaasa, Finland outpatients (Jan–Feb 1996)

Dimension	Weight	Perceptions	Expectations	Gap
Tangibles	0.18	5.64	6.03	-0.38
Reliability	0.21	5.51	6.04	-0.54
Responsiveness	0.20	5.73	6.12	-0.39
Assurance	0.22	5.83	6.23	-0.40
Empathy	0.19	5.74	6.08	-0.35
Weighted averages (n = 135)		5.72	6.14	-0.41

The Utility of the SERVQUAL Model

The SERVQUAL methodology goes some way towards meeting the objection, noted before, that the issues raised in any instrument inevitably reflect the interests of the producers rather than the ultimate consumers of services, including health. The framers of the SERVQUAL methodology (Parasuraman, Zeithaml and Berry, 1985, 1988; Zeithaml, Parasuraman and Berry, 1990) took pains to ensure that the elements of the instrument they devised were derived from a series of focused interviews and were then subjected to detailed factor analysis to discern the elements of the SERVQUAL scale. The standardized nature of the questions means that the instrument is particularly useful in comparative studies, such as between different industries, societies or time periods. The essential simplicity of the approach, combined with the fact that it specifically relativizes the context of satisfaction by addressing the issue of prior expectations, may be an explanation for its extensive use as a quality metric for service-type industries. However, two fundamental objections can be made which may severely limit the potential of this type of approach – one on the conceptual level and the other on the methodology actually deployed.

The first of these objections relates to the 'split' which is discerned between expectations on the one hand and service delivery on the other. The weight given to the measurement of expectations implies that consumers (or patients in this instance) approach their encounters with medical professionals with a set of clearly articulated expectations. However, it is useful to see patient interactions with clinicians not as a series of one-off transactions but as a series of episodes linked together into a *trajectory*. The concept of a disease trajectory is evident in standard medical practice but in social scientific terms the notion of trajectory approaches the transactions in a more dynamic way, such that expectations of the next encounter are likely to be a function of previous encounters. Typically, when patients present themselves to clinical staff with a problem that requires resolution, they are entering into a series of transactions which may involve dozens of different professionals extending over several years or, indeed, a lifetime. One of the most typical trajectories might be as follows:

initial consultation – diagnostic tests – inpatient treatment – outpatient follow-up

and in such a trajectory (particularly in the case of inpatient treatment within hospitals) an individual, and the data relating to the individual, is processed by many personnel working in diverse occupational domains (manual occupations such as portering, clerical and administrative staff, medical, nursing and paramedical staff and so on). To attempt to capture the intricacies of such dynamics by the use of a single snapshot-type instrument would appear to be overambitious. It has been observed several times before that expectations might not be fully formed at the point of first contact with clinical staff and may be free-floating or even epiphenomenal, in that expectations start to arise out of the dynamics of the interactions with clinical staff (Locker and Dunt, 1978; Avis, Bond and Arthur, 1995; Linder-Pelz, 1982). Measures of patient satisfaction are typically frozen in one point of time and do not (perhaps cannot) acknowledge the importance of trajectories in the measurement of satisfaction.

The Use and Abuse of Rating Scales

A conventional 'orthodoxy' follows Stevens (1946) categorization of scales into nominal, ordinal, interval and ratio. As Blalock (1979) explains:

> It is important to recognise that an ordinal level of measurement does not supply any information about the **MAGNITUDE** of the differences between elements. We know only that A is greater than B but cannot say how much greater. Nor can we say that the difference between A and B is less than that between C and D. We therefore cannot add or subtract differences except in a very restricted sense. For example if we had the following relationships:

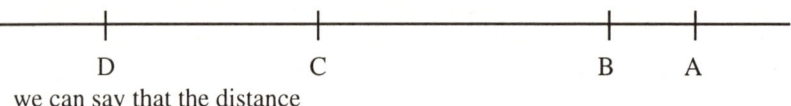

> we can say that the distance

$$\overline{AD} = \overline{AB} + \overline{BC} + \overline{CD}$$

but we cannot attempt to compare the distances $\overline{AB}$ and $\overline{CD}$. In other words, when we translate order relations into mathematical operations, we cannot, in general, use the usual operations of addition, subtraction, multiplication and division. We can, however, use the operations 'greater than' and 'less than' if these prove useful ... (p. 17).

One of the dangers of 'cookbook statistics' is the tendency to oversimplify the criteria and problems involved in making basic decisions in data analysis. It is impossible to over-emphasise the important point that, in any using any statistical technique, one must be aware of the underlying assumptions that the procedure requires. In the context of the present discussion, one of the first questions that must always be asked concerns the level of measurement that can legitimately be assumed (p. 24).

An alternative view is held by many behavioural scientists and by some statisticians (e.g., Anderson, 1972). As Lord (1972), in an entertaining article observes, the statistical test can hardly be cognizant of the empirical meaning of the numbers with which it deals: 'Since the numbers don't remember where they came from, they always behave the same way, regardless'.

On a more pragmatic level, Anderson argues, if the difference between parametric and ran-order tests was not great insofar as significance level and power are concerned, then only the versatility of parametric statistics meets the needs of everyday (psychological) research.

The argument, then, is often conducted between those who follow the 'conventionalist' position of Stevens (1946), Blalock (1979), Siegel and Castellan (1988) and the majority of textbook writers on the one hand, and a more 'pragmatic' school on the other, who would maintain that the assumptions about scale type can probably be relaxed quite greatly without too much violence being done to the integrity of the data. In the case of psychological research, it could be that other sources of error (e.g. slightly different phrasing of questions) assume much more significance as sources of error than arguments over scale type.

One of the most recent and informed papers in this debate is by Hand (1996) who draws distinctions between the *representational, operational* and *classical* measurement paradigms. *Representational* theory assigns numbers to objects to model their relationships. *Operational* theory, on the other hand, assigns numbers according to some consistent measurement systems and represents objects as congruent with the measurement system. Finally, *classical* theory involves the discovery of relationships between different quantities of a given attribute. There is, therefore, an assumption that there is a deeper reality which it is the aim of the analyst to discover – *classical* because traces of this approach can be found in the writings of Aristotle and of Euclid. The choice of test, therefore, is not so much a technical matter as a philosophical one – it depends on the nature of the model and the philosophy of science held by the investigator.

In the case of a rating scale attempting to measure satisfaction (*pace* SERVQUAL) then it is possible that we could adopt one of the following positions:

1   the measures are essentially ordinal. Whatever point on the scale is adopted, then we can assume that we can make statements which assign a degree of ordering but we cannot get involved in the mathematical operations of subtraction of one measure from another. So statements such as satisfaction = perceptions - expectations (the core of SERVQUAL) are illegitimate;

2   already not strictly forming a series of continuous data, a scale such as seven point SERVQUAL scale inviting agreement/disagreement with a series of propositions can, for practical purposes, be assumed to be relatively monotonic. In the absence of evidence to indicate a large degree of skewness in the data, then the conventional parametric tests can be deployed, as it has been shown that such tests can actually tolerate fairly large violations of the assumptions of normality of underlying distributions before they lose validity.

An alternative approach might be to follow the offered by Kind et al. (1993), in which probabilities in a questionnaire are derived from cumulative frequency distributions of the responses and then converted into the corresponding z-scores based on a normal distribution.

Some authors such as Lodge (1981) have deployed the concept of *magnitude scaling* in which an underlying scale is inferred from the magnitudes associated with a series of common adjectives (e.g. good, very good, excellent) which respondents have been asked to quantify.

The Quantitative Analysis of Open-ended Responses

A more obvious way to measure the distribution of patient responses is to capture responses by the use of the most open-ended questions possible and then chart the distribution of the responses. The following example is drawn from a qualitative investigation of paediatric outreach clinics, conducted by the author (n = 64). The overall sample statistics are shown in Table 5.4.

Table 5.4   'What would you say was a *good* clinic?'

	Value	No.	Cum_n	%	Cumpct	Barchart	
Friendly staff	1	22	22	27.16	27.16	■■■■■■	22
Good consultation	2	21	43	25.93	53.09	■■■■■	21
No long waiting time	3	17	60	20.99	74.07	■■■■	17
Nothing in particular	4	11	71	13.58	87.65	■■■	11
Facilities for children	5	5	76	6.17	93.83	■	5
Access, convenience	6	3	79	3.70	97.53	■	3
Better than ??? hospital	7	2	81	2.47	100.00	■	2

What Makes for a 'Good' Clinic Session?

The two factors mentioned that accounted for more than all other factors combined were the overall friendliness of the staff and the quality of the communication with the consultant. Parents were evidently anxious to get a diagnosis of the symptoms which had led them to the clinic in the first place. Representative comments are:

> Dr ___ makes the child feel relaxed and not agitated. The doctor is always very friendly.

> A 'good' clinic is when you are listened to and the doctor is interested in you. Then, you do not feel the clinic is a waste of time.

> When the doctor tries to explain things to you and talks things through. This can help to alleviate my worries …

Some patients referred to the totality of the transactions that they held with clinic staff:

[A good clinic is ...] the helpfulness of the staff. Nothing is too much trouble for them. You cannot really fault them at all ...

After the friendliness of the staff and the communication with the consultant, the absence of a long waiting time was the third most-mentioned factor:

[A good clinic is] one that is easier for the children in the area ... it's easier than [central hospital] where you usually have to wait a long time.

(NB: 64 respondents mentioned 81 factors as some respondents mentioned more than one factor.)

Here, standard content analysis is used to measure the different types of responses. These are then diagrammed using any statistical software package (in this case, MICROSTATS). The virtue of this approach is that patients are allowed to 'speak for themselves'. The analyst can show the typicality of responses by using conventional statistical graphing measures whilst the choice of quotations can help to 'bring alive' the nature of the data collected.

Accountability in the 'New' NHS

There is now increasing evidence that a heavy reliance upon quantitative measures of quality such as activity rates and waiting times fails adequately to address some of the more fundamental questions such as patient expectations and perceptions. Even when performance indicators are couched in quantitative terms, they are rarely transmitted to front-line staff (Goddard, 1997). A recent survey of health authorities and trusts (Wakeley, 1997) indicated a serious commitment to quality – indeed 49 per cent of health authorities would accept a reduction in activity levels for a demonstrable improvement in quality. However, it is possible to incorporate the views of the users into healthcare planning and provision, long advocated by patient advocates such as Rigge (1997) and demonstrated in initiatives such as consumer-led audit in Lothian (Stevenson and Hegarty, 1994).

An instrument such as SERVQUAL could play its part in establishing the particular gaps between service provision and patients' experiences of such services. Its standardized nature and the fact that it has been utilized in a wide variety of studies across many different service sector industries could help to avoid the difficulties associated with the traditional patient satisfaction survey which has often been criticized in the past as being too 'producer-oriented'. At the same time, it is important that the patients help to shape the *agenda* of the measurement of quality issues . This, in turn, implies that health service managers and clinicians need to develop skills in the collection, interpretation and analysis of qualitative data to supplement more quantitative measures which, it could be argued, have traditionally been accorded a greater weight than is strictly merited.

Conclusions

The traditional instruments for the analysis of patient satisfaction are still being deployed, despite the many criticisms that have been made of them. This chapter indicates the possibilities and the problems associated with deploying a conventional and widely known method of gap analysis such as SERVQUAL. The chapter concludes by indicating that it is quite possible to collect and to analyse data which is consumer- rather than producer-led and to deploy some of the tools of quantitative analysis associated with more conventional approaches in this area. It is possible that more work needs to be undertaken which marries together a more ethnographic or patient-centred approaches in which patients 'speak for themselves' with a degree of quantitative analysis which indicates the typicality of the responses made.

References

Anderson, N.H. (1972), 'Scales and Statistics: Parametric and non-parametric' in R.E. Kirk (ed.), *Statistical Issues: A Reader for the Behavioural Sciences*, Brooks/Cole, Monterrey.

Avis, M., Bond, M. and Arthur, A. (1995), 'Satisfying solution? A review of some unresolved issues in the measurement of patient satisfaction', *Journal of Advanced Nursing*, 22, pp. 316–22.

Baker, R. and Whitfield, M. (1992), 'Measuring Patient Satisfaction: A test of construct validity', *Quality in Health Care*, 1 (2), pp. 104–9.

Bamford, C. and Jacoby, A. (1992), 'Development of patient satisfaction questionnaires: I. Methodological issues', *Quality in Health Care*, 1 (3), pp. 153–7.

Batalden, P. and Nelson, E. (1990), 'Hospital Quality: Patient, Physician and Employee Judgements', *International Journal of Health Care Quality Assurance*, 3 (4), pp. 7–17.

Batchelor, C., Owens, D.J., Read, M. and Bloor, M. (1994), 'Patient Satisfaction Studies: Methodology, Management and Consumer Evaluation', *International Journal of Health Care Quality Assurance*, 7 (7), pp. 22–30.

Blalock, H. M. (1979), *Social Statistics*, revised 2nd edn, McGraw-Hill Kogakusha, London.

Carr-Hill, R. (1992), 'The measurement of patient satisfaction', *Journal of Public Health Medicine*, 14 (3), pp. 236–49.

Carr-Hill, R., Humphries, K. and McIver, S. (1987), *Wolverhampton: a picture of health*, mimeograph, York, Centre for Health Economics.

College of Health (1994), *Consumer Audit Guidelines*, College of Health, London.

DHSS (1983), *Enquiry into NHS Management* (The Griffiths Report), HMSO, London.

Eccles, M., Jacoby, A. and Bamford, C. (1992) 'Development of patient satisfaction questionnaires: II. Collaboration in practice', *Quality in Health Care*, 1 (3), pp. 158–60.

Ellis, R. and Whittington, D. (1994), 'Health Care Quality Assurance: Techniques and Approaches', *Public Money and Management*, 14 (2), pp. 23–9.

Evason, E. and Whittington, D. (1991), 'Patient Satisfaction Studies: Problems and Implications Explored in a Pilot Study in Northern Ireland', *Health Education Journal*, 50 (2), pp. 73–7.

Fitzpatrick, R. (1991a), 'Surveys of Patient Satisfaction: I–Important General Considerations', *British Medical Journal*, 302, pp. 887–9.

Fitzpatrick, R. (1991b), 'Surveys of Patient Satisfaction: II–Designing a Questionnaire and Conducting a Survey', *British Medical Journal*, 302, pp. 1129–32.

Goddard, M. (1998), 'All quiet on the front line', *Health Service Journal*, 14 May, pp. 24–6.

Hand, D.J. (1996), 'Statistics and the theory of measurement', *Journal of the Royal Statistical Society*, Series A, 159 (3), pp. 445–92.

Kind, P., Leese, B., Cameron, I. and Carpenter, J. (1993), 'Quantifying Quality – Measuring Quality in the Provision of Health Care' in M. Malek, P. Vacani, J. Rasquinha and P. Davey (eds), *Managerial Issues in the Reformed NHS*, John Wiley & Sons, Chichester.

Linder-Pelz, S. (1982), 'Toward a theory of patient satisfaction', *Social Science and Medicine*, 16, p. 577.

Locker, D. and Dunt, D. (1978), 'Theoretical and methodological issues in sociological studies of consumer satisfaction with medical care', *Social Science and Medicine*, 12, pp. 283–92.

Lodge, M. (1981) *Magnitude Scaling*, Sage University Paper Series on Quantitative Applications in the Social Sciences No. 25, Sage, Beverly Hills.

Lord, F.M. (1972), 'On the statistical treatment of football numbers' in R.E. Kirk (ed.), *Statistical Issues: A Reader for the Behavioural Sciences*, Brooks/Cole, Monterrey.

NHS Management Executive (1992), *Local Voices – The Views of Local People in Purchasing for Health*, EL(92)1, January.

Parasuraman, A., Zeithaml, V. and Berry, L. (1985), 'A Conceptual Model of Service Quality and its implications for Future Research', *Journal of Marketing*, 49 (Fall), pp. 41–50.

Parasuraman, A., Zeithaml, V. and Berry, L. (1988), 'SERVQUAL: A Multiple-Item Scale for Measuring Perceptions of Service Quality', *Journal of Retailing*, 64, pp. 12–40.

Rigge, M. (1995), 'Does public opinion matter ? (Yes/No/Don't know)', *Health Service Journal*, 7 September, pp. 26–7.

Rigge, M. (1997), 'Keeping the customer satisfied', *Health Service Journal*, 30 October, pp. 24–7.

Scott, A. and Smith, R. (1994), 'Keeping the Customer Satisfied: Issues in the Interpretation and Use of Patient Satisfaction Surveys', *International Journal for Quality in Health Care*, 6 (4), pp. 353–9.

Siegel, S. and Castellan, N.J. (1988), *Nonparametric Statistics*, 2nd edn, McGraw-Hill, New York.

Stevens, S.S. (1946), 'On the theory of scales of measurement', *Science*, 103, pp. 677–80.

Stevenson, R. and Hegarty, M. (1994), 'In the picture', *Health Services Journal*, 24 November, pp. 22–4.

Wakeley, M. (1997), 'Quality Commitment', *Health Service Journal*, 7 August 1997, pp. 28–9.

Zeithaml, V., Parasuraman, A. and Berry, L. (1990), *Delivering Service Quality*, Free Press, New York.

Appendix 1 SERVQUAL questionnaire

Based on your experiences as a patient in a hospital or clinic, please think about the kind of hospital or clinic that would deliver excellent quality of service. Think about the kind of hospital or clinic in which you would like to receive treatment. Please show the extent to which you think such a hospital or clinic would possess the feature described by each statement. If you feel a feature is *not at all essential* for excellent hospitals/clinics such as the one you have in mind, circle the number 1. If you feel a feature is *absolutely essential* for excellent hospitals/clinics, circle 7. If your feelings are less strong, circle one of the numbers in the middle. There are no right or wrong answers – all we are interested in is the number that truly reflects your feelings regarding hospitals/clinics that would deliver excellent quality of service.

		Strongly Disagree						Strongly Agree
1.	Excellent hospitals/clinics will have modern looking equipment.	1	2	3	4	5	6	7
2.	The physical facilities at excellent hospitals will be visually appealing.	1	2	3	4	5	6	7
3.	Personnel at excellent hospitals/clinics will be neat in appearance.	1	2	3	4	5	6	7
4.	Materials associated with the service (such as pamphlets or statements) will be visually appealing in an excellent hospital/clinic.	1	2	3	4	5	6	7
5.	When excellent hospitals/clinics promise to do something by a certain time they will do so.	1	2	3	4	5	6	7
6.	When a patient has a problem, excellent hospitals/clinics will show a sincere interest in solving it.	1	2	3	4	5	6	7

	Strongly Disagree					Strongly Agree

7. Excellent hospitals/clinics will get things right the first time. 1 2 3 4 5 6 7

8. Excellent hospitals/clinics will provide their services at the time they promise to do so. 1 2 3 4 5 6 7

9. Excellent hospitals/clinics will insist on error-free records. 1 2 3 4 5 6 7

10. Personnel in excellent hospitals/clinics will tell patients exactly when services will be performed. 1 2 3 4 5 6 7

11. Personnel in excellent hospitals/clinics will give prompt service to patients. 1 2 3 4 5 6 7

12. Personnel in excellent hospitals/clinics will always be willing to help patients. 1 2 3 4 5 6 7

13. Personnel in excellent hospitals/clinics will never be too busy to respond to patients' requests. 1 2 3 4 5 6 7

14. The behaviour of personnel in excellent hospitals/clinics will instil confidence in patients. 1 2 3 4 5 6 7

15. Patients of excellent hospitals/clinics will feel safe in their dealings with the hospital/clinic. 1 2 3 4 5 6 7

16. Personnel in excellent hospitals/clinics will be consistently courteous with patients. 1 2 3 4 5 6 7

	Strongly Disagree					**Strongly Agree**	
17. Personnel in excellent hospitals/clinics will have the knowledge to answer patients' questions.	1	2	3	4	5	6	7
18. Excellent hospitals/clinics will give patients individual attention.	1	2	3	4	5	6	7
19. Excellent hospitals/clinics will have operating hours convenient to all their patients.	1	2	3	4	5	6	7
20. Excellent hospitals/clinics will have staff who give patients personal attention.	1	2	3	4	5	6	7
21. Excellent hospitals/clinics will have the patients' best interests at heart.	1	2	3	4	5	6	7
22. The personnel of excellent hospitals/clinics will understand the specific needs of their patients.	1	2	3	4	5	6	7

Listed below are five features pertaining to hospitals/clinics and the service they offer. We would like to know how important each of these features is to *you* when you evaluate the service offered by a hospital or clinic. Please allocate a total of 100 points among the five features *according to how important each feature is to you* – the more important a feature is to you, the more points you should allocate to it. Please ensure that the points you allocate to the five features add up to 100.

1. The appearance of the hospital/clinic's physical facilities, equipment, personnel and communication materials.   _____ points

2. The hospital/clinic's ability to perform the promised service dependably and accurately.   _____ points

3. The hospital/clinic's willingness to help patients and provide
   a prompt service.   _____ points

4. The knowledge and courtesy of the hospital/clinic personnel
   and their ability to convey trust and confidence.   _____ points

5. The caring, individualized attention the hospital/clinic
   provides its patients.   _____ points

TOTAL points allocated   100 points

Which one feature of the above five is most important to you?   _____
(Please enter the feature's number)

Which feature is second most important to you?   _____

Which feature is least important to you?   _____

The following set of statements relate to your feelings about the hospital/
clinic you have attended. For each statement, please show the extent to which
you believe the hospital/clinic has the feature described by the statement.
Once again, circling a 1. means that you strongly disagree that the hospital/
clinic you have attended has this feature and circling a 7. means that you
strongly agree. You may circle any of the numbers in the middle that show
how strong your feelings are. There are no right or wrong answers – all we
are interested in is a number that best shows your perceptions about the hospital/
clinic which has treated you.

	Strongly Disagree						Strongly Agree
1. The hospital/clinic has modern-looking equipment.	1	2	3	4	5	6	7
2. The physical facilities in the hospital/clinic are visually appealing.	1	2	3	4	5	6	7

	Strongly Disagree					Strongly Agree	

3. Personnel in the hospital/clinic are neat in appearance.　1　2　3　4　5　6　7

4. Materials associated with the service (such as pamphlets or statements) are visually appealing.　1　2　3　4　5　6　7

5. When the hospital/clinic promises to do something by a certain time it does so.　1　2　3　4　5　6　7

6. When you have a problem, the hospitals/clinic shows a sincere interest in solving it.　1　2　3　4　5　6　7

7. The hospital/clinic gets things right the first time.　1　2　3　4　5　6　7

8. The hospital/clinic provides its services at the time it promises to do so.　1　2　3　4　5　6　7

9. The hospital/clinic insists on error-free records.　1　2　3　4　5　6　7

10. The personnel in the hospital/clinic tell you exactly when services will be performed.　1　2　3　4　5　6　7

11. Personnel in the hospital/clinic give you prompt service.　1　2　3　4　5　6　7

12. Personnel in the hospital/clinic are always willing to help you.　1　2　3　4　5　6　7

	Strongly Disagree						Strongly Agree
13. Personnel in the hospital/clinic are never be too busy to respond to your requests.	1	2	3	4	5	6	7
14. The behaviour of personnel in the hospital/ clinic instils confidence in you.	1	2	3	4	5	6	7
15. You feel safe in your dealings with the hospital/clinic.	1	2	3	4	5	6	7
16. Personnel in the hospital/clinic are consistently courteous with you.	1	2	3	4	5	6	7
17. Personnel in the hospital/clinic have the knowledge to answer your questions.	1	2	3	4	5	6	7
18. The hospital/clinic gives you individual attention.	1	2	3	4	5	6	7
19. The hospital/clinic has operating hours convenient to all its patients.	1	2	3	4	5	6	7
20. The hospital/clinic has personnel who give you personal attention.	1	2	3	4	5	6	7
21. The hospital/clinic has your best interests at heart.	1	2	3	4	5	6	7
22. The personnel of the hospital/clinic understand your specific needs.	1	2	3	4	5	6	7

Thank you for the time you have spent in completing this questionnaire. The results will help us to provide you with the best possible service in the future.

Appendix 2 SERVQUAL procedures

Dimensions

Statements	**1–4**	Tangibles
Statements	**5–9**	Reliability
Statements	**10–13**	Responsiveness
Statements	**14–17**	Assurance
Statements	**18–22**	Empathy

Procedures

1.   Compute the 'gap' for each statement pair for each consumer.

   SERVQUAL score = Perceptions Score – Expectations Score

2.   Compute the dimensions scores for each respondent by averaging the gap score over the relevant number of statements (either **4** or **5** statements).

3.   Derive **SERVQUAL** respondent's scores in the following way:

   Unweighted scores Sum dimensions and divide by 5

Weighted scores	Tangibles *	(Tangibles Weight/100)	+
	Reliability *	(Reliability Weight/100)	+
	Responsiveness *	(Responsiveness Weight/100)	+
	Assurance *	(Assurance Weight/100)	+
	Empathy *	(Empathy Weight/100).	

4.   Derive total **SERVQUAL** scores by totalling the scores and dividing by **N** of respondents.

Note: a computer program to automate these procedures (any IBM PC compatible) is available from the author.

6 Managing Clinical Audit: Diagnosing the Problems and Designing Solutions

GAIL JOHNSTON,[1] HUW T.O. DAVIES,[2] IAIN K. CROMBIE,[3]
ELIZABETH M. ALDER[3] AND ANDREW R. MILLARD [4]

1 *Department of General Practice, Queen's University of Belfast*
2 *Department of Management, University of St Andrews*
3 *Department of Epidemiology and Public Health, Ninewells Medical School, Dundee*
4 *Scottish Clinical Audit Resource Centre, University of Glasgow*

Introduction

Recent governmental interest in audit dates from the publication of a 1989 White Paper on the NHS (Department of Health, 1989). Commitment to audit was reiterated in 1998 in the latest White Paper produced by the incoming Labour government (Department of Health, 1997). Trust Chief Executives now have responsibility for the effectiveness of the services they provide (Black, 1998). Despite this, almost a decade after its formal introduction, few of the anticipated benefits of audit have been realized and critics are questioning its value and continued government investment (Fulton, 1996; Maynard, 1991; Mooney and Ryan, 1992). The majority of audit activity remains haphazard and unfocused with few obvious benefits to patient care (Miles et al., 1996; Walshe and Coles, 1995). In addition, there is still substantial dissent among clinicians about its usefulness (Thomson and Barton, 1994) and much confusion as to how to carry it out (Nolan and Scott, 1993; Miles et al., 1996).

The incoming Labour government has made quality the centrepiece of its reforms (Secretary of State for Health, 1998). Although the new strategy makes much of increased central control through a wide range of performance indicators, it also spells out the need for a reinvigorated audit programme

Managing Quality: Strategic Issues in Health Care Management, H.T.O. Davies, M. Tavakoli, M. Malek, A.R. Neilson (eds), Ashgate Publishing Ltd, 1999.

contained within a new framework for clinical governance (Davies and Mannion, 1999). If audit is to deliver on some of the government's quality promises, then the reasons for audit's chequered history need to be explored and addressed. For all that clinical audit is a clinical responsibility, the context within which audit takes places and the institutional arrangements for its encouragement are also partly a managerial responsibility (Dunning et al., 1998).

This chapter explores and evaluates health care professionals' experiences of audit. It does so with the aim of uncovering managerial issues that, if addressed, would foster successful care-improving audit projects. The material is arranged in three sections. First we describe what health professionals themselves see as the role and aims of audit, and we explore their perceptions of its benefits and drawbacks. Second, we explain the difficulties that would-be auditors face in conducting successful studies. Finally, the key managerial responses are identified and discussed. Throughout the text we draw on an extensive published literature and make use of direct quotes gathered during a study which interviewed health care professionals in Scotland about their experiences with audit (Johnston et al., 1998).

Audit from the Health Professionals' Perspective

Many (but by no means all) clinicians[1] have been enthusiastic participants in clinical audit from its inception. Identifying the reasons for this enthusiasm (and reasons for its absence) may help identify how the organizational culture could be modified to foster more positive attitudes. Surveys of clinicians report several perceived benefits as a consequence of taking part in audit (Penney et al., 1995). These range from positive changes in the quality of service provided to patients (Pringle et al., 1994; Willmot et al., 1995; National Audit Office, 1994; Cooper and French, 1993; Toy, 1994), to professional benefits such as enhanced communication with colleagues and improved personal satisfaction and knowledge (Eccles et al., 1995; Johnson, 1994; Watkins and King, 1996; Lewis and Combes 1996). Of particular importance seems to be the detailed insight into personal practice that audit brings, and the scope this provides for personal learning: 'We were able to look critically at ourselves. People will only learn if they are provided with evidence which compares them badly to other people'.[2]

Changing and improving health care is at the heart of audit and yet those participating in audit projects also identify a range of other substantial benefits, such as improved professional status among colleagues, a greater understanding of roles between disciplines and better chances of promotion (Robinson, 1996b). Thus clinicians may use audit as a means of justifying new roles or raising the status of an established team or discipline:

> I was aware through the literature that non-health staff and even some primary carers and acute staff were saying ... what exactly do they do? ... We had to be better at actually evidencing and being clearer about exactly what we were doing and why were doing it.

Audit is also sometimes used as a means of career advancement:

> I wanted to get a paper. For a training grade that's usually the reason for doing something like this – to get a publication.

Thus clinicians have a variety of motives for conducting audit which are much broader than simply improving care. Improving legitimacy, status and career prospects are powerful motives which health care managers could use directly to encourage more active participation in audit. There is no reason why meeting some of these objectives could not be married to the key objective of improving the quality of patient care.

Of course, not all clinicians are well disposed towards audit or are convinced of its benefits. Many remain sceptical that it improves the quality of care (Kerrison et al. 1993; Sellu 1996). Understanding these perceptions too may provide guidance on how such attitudes may be changed.

Audit is seen by some clinicians as both time wasting and a distraction from patient care (Smith et al. 1992; Davison and Smith 1993; Barton and Spencer 1994; Webb et al., 1991). Others see it simply as boring, and a burdensome task that has to be endured – rather than an inherent and integral part of clinical practice (Greenhalgh 1992; Sherwood 1992; Farrell 1995). Thus for all those who are enthusiastic about audit, others are disinterested and unmotivated:

> If I had a couple of spare hours I'd rather go to the bank or play some golf rather than say oh I've got two hours it's 3 o'clock I better work, I'll do some audit till 5 ....

Clinicians are also sometimes suspicious about the underlying motives for audit. For example, they may be concerned that audit activities may lead to a reduction in clinical ownership (Foster et al., 1996), increase professional marginalization (Kerrison et al., 1993), or prompt litigation (Webb and Harvey, 1992). In addition, the multidisciplinary aspects of audit lead to fears that it may undermine relationships between professional groups (McKenna, 1995). Junior staff in particular report feeling intimidated, ridiculed and threatened by audit activities which single them out for unfair criticism (Black and Thompson, 1993; Firth-Cozens and Storer, 1992).

Negative experiences of audit will certainly dissuade clinicians from further active and committed involvement. However, the wide range of perceived benefits offers the opportunity to engage clinicians by addressing explicitly their multiple motivations. The difficulty for health care managers lies in constructing a supportive environment within which audit can flourish without encroaching on sensitivities about clinical autonomy. This suggests the need for development of a truly participative quality strategy at a local level in order to break down old attitudes and instil a common understanding about the aims and processes of audit. The approach should recognize the multiplicity of motivations and benefits of participation in audit and should directly address clinicians' fears.

Conducting Audit: Pitfalls and Problems

Carrying out audit seems deceptively simple: identify a problem area; set some explicit standards; collect some data to assess current practice and compliance with those standards; then instigate changes to improve care (Crombie and Davies, 1992; Crombie et al., 1993; Crombie and Davies, 1994). However, numerous studies report that clinicians have trouble with all of these different aspects.

Although some audits are carried out single-handedly, most projects require a collaborative effort. Even in the early stages problems often arise. Difficulties with group dynamics can result when members fail to gel effectively and differences between individuals impede their effective functioning (Eccles et al., 1995; Robinson, 1996a; Buttery et al., 1995a). There may be a failure to agree on the delegation of tasks and often there is a lack of clear understanding between members of different disciplines about the boundaries of each other's roles (Eccles et al., 1995). These difficulties are often made worse by the physical problems involved in bringing a group of busy staff together in a mutually convenient place and time which are protected from interruptions (Eccles et al., 1996; Kerrison et al., 1993). Interviews with recent auditors suggest that groups work best when members share a common goal and equal commitment to the topic of the audit:

> Everybody was signed up to it. Everybody could see it was a good idea.

Unsurprisingly, group work suffers when the commitment of members is unequal or wanes, when members have different views, or when there is an unequal sharing of tasks and a lack of clear objectives. As a result decision making becomes protracted, tasks often fall to one or only a few members of the group and sometimes groups disband altogether:

> There were lots of ideas about what to look at but we couldn't agree on the most important.

Once organized and ready to go, audit groups often find that the surface simplicity of audit hides a deeper complexity which they are ill-equipped to tackle (Foster et al., 1996; Lough et al., 1995; Willmot et al., 1995). As a result, projects are often poorly designed (Firth-Cozens and Storer, 1992; Willmot et al., 1995; Davies et al., 1995) and badly executed (Tabendeh and Thompson, 1995). The learning curve is steep and opportunities to be misled are many: as one clinician commented:

> I didn't know what questions to ask to get the information I wanted. I did it back to front really. I was guided by the technology. There was a lot of pain and suffering involved.

Perhaps through blissful ignorance, many clinicians embark on overly ambitious projects that are beyond their level of expertise. A telling remark from a newly enlightened clinician encapsulates this:

> We should have started small and got bigger instead of starting big and collapsing.

Clinicians' lack of expertise may be exacerbated by a scarcity of support staff to provide them with the extra help they require (Buttery et al., 1994; Webb and Harvey, 1994; Karran et al., 1993). This lack is deeply felt:

> As far as I'm aware they (the audit department) have made it quite clear that they didn't have a lot of staff. … It would be absolutely fantastic if they could say oh great that's fine that's the form you want filled in. We'll get the case notes dug out, we'll fill all the forms out for you and then we'll get back and discuss how to crunch the statistics. That would be wonderful.

In addition, even when local human resources are available, the individuals may lack experience and skills. Teachers of audit and audit support staff are themselves sometimes inadequately trained in appropriate audit methods, and thus face the same steep learning curve as those they are intended to help (Hopkins, 1996; Spencer, 1992).

One of the biggest difficulties in achieving effective audit lies in changing clinical practice even in the face of manifest shortcomings. Even those projects that are well executed may founder because of poorly developed relationships with those in authority who can enforce change (Robinson, 1996a). Poor relationships with management may also lead to organizational barriers that can obstruct the process of audit (Webb and Harvey, 1994; Lord and Littlejohns, 1994).

The views of managers and clinicians often differ with each side bringing different agendas to the audit arena (Smith et al., 1992; Thomson et al., 1996; Karran et al., 1993; Berger, 1998). As a result clinicians are sometimes unclear about who can sanction the implementation of changes especially if they are beyond clinicians' immediate area of responsibility (Sellu, 1996). On a wider scale, the implementation of changes may be further obstructed by managers' reluctance to make changes that have financial implications (ibid.). Clinicians regularly bemoan managers' lack of commitment to follow projects through:

> Unless I get support from other boards [Health Authorities – purchasers] or from external sources, the thing will just crumble. ... it is disappointing that at the end of the audit there really isn't the weight of support from the Trust.

This lack of acknowledgement from managers can also make clinicians question the value of audit and can undermine their support for further audit activity:

> What ward staff feel is that you hear people waffling on about audit but get no encouragement to do it from management ... When morale in the ward is so low it doesn't take much to say I can't be bothered doing it.

Underlying many of these issues is the recurrent theme of inadequate resources. By far the greatest barrier to carrying out audit, as perceived by clinicians, is a lack of dedicated time (Davison and Smith, 1993; Karran et al., 1993; Robinson, 1996a; Baker et al., 1995). As a result clinicians are forced to juggle audit activities with the conflicting demands of patient care (National Audit Office, 1994). This problem is exacerbated by a lack of supportive mechanisms to facilitate clinicians' involvement in audit such as adequate funding, dedicated support staff and good quality information systems (Firth-Cozens and Storer, 1992; National Audit Office, 1994). Consequently, many clinicians spend much of their own free time in order to undertake audit projects:

> The onus is definitely moving more and more towards it's more important to write a good story than to give the care. Everything is designed to take you off the shop floor ... If I've got monthly stats to do and staff assessments to do and if you come along and say will you throw an audit in the middle of that I'll say I don't have the time. It is a deterrent. It definitely is off putting.

The multitude of difficulties facing even well-motivated auditors suggests plenty of scope for managerial action. Possible responses are discussed in the next section.

Responding to the Problems

That clinical audit should be an activity under clinical control is rarely in dispute. Yet upholding clinical autonomy in this regard can sometimes seem like abandonment of any obligation to develop an appropriate infrastructure, provide adequate resources and develop a supportive quality culture. Given the range and diversity of problems outlined in the previous sections, concerted action, jointly conceived between mangers and clinicians, may have much to offer.

Studies of medical and clinical audit programmes have identified many factors that facilitate successful audit (Walshe, 1995; Lervy et al., 1994; Grol and Wensing, 1995; Chambers et al., 1995; Hearnshaw et al., 1994). These include a climate where audit activity is acknowledged by management and peers as an appropriate use of clinicians' time, a well planned and supported audit programme, and protected time to relieve the pressure on clinicians' workload. In addition, effective training programmes, simplifying access to funding, and improved methods of data collection can all contribute. Attention to each of these can stimulate both more audit activity and more effective audit projects (Rumsey et al., 1996a, 1996b; Bennett and Coles, 1996; Buttery et al., 1995b). Interviews with the Scottish sample support and augment these findings and suggest that these are practical ways in which management can work to operationalize these factors.

Evaluations of audit programmes emphasize the importance of a shared audit culture between management and clinicians to ensure its success. Yet this culture is not a reality for many health care professionals. The importance of audit to managers should be recognized by publicizing findings from local studies through newsletters and regular symposia. Reports from projects should be recorded on a central register and managers should make more effort to acknowledge these and act on the findings. In addition, the benefits to individuals of conducting audit in terms of career and professional development could be more widely addressed.

Putting in place a supportive network of skilled audit support would also convince care staff that audit is a worthwhile use of their clinical time. These support services must be openly accessible to all levels and disciplines equally. Clinicians' comments, however, also suggest that support must be tailored to their requirements. While some clinicians want to hand over all audit related tasks to the audit department others would prefer to retain ownership by doing much of the audit themselves:

> Asking for audit department support would have expanded time again because they would have rejigged it to suit themselves and we didn't want that.

Conversely, there are those who would not contemplate doing audit without the support of a facilitator. Of course, clinicians need to know what is available to them before they can decide on the level of input they require. Overall, the key role of the audit facilitator needs greater recognition and Trust audit committees should have an audit programme for facilitators to implement. Trusts should assess whether more audit support staff should be employed to provide hands-on help. Whenever possible facilitators should take an active role in the planning, day-to-day management and analysis of projects.

As many otherwise enthusiastic clinicians lack the necessary skills to design and implement effective audits, this is an obvious target for managerial action. As with audit department support, however, it is apparent that the content of training courses should vary with the needs of individual staff groups. While some clinicians do want more extended training, most appear to want short sharp courses that introduce them to the mechanics of audit or refresh previous training experiences:

> I could have been better trained. You learn a lot from doing the thing. I don't think any more formal theory would be useful. We need some way to make audit part of nurse training – make it subtler for longer all the way down.

I think there is a danger that people train for training's sake whereas if you had a specific task I would certainly take up the offer of more training. I worry generally about training that people are not task orientated enough.

Some of the skills needed for audit are those of the specialist and it would not be sensible to attempt to teach these skills to everyone. The availability of expert advisers to augment the support of the audit department and staff training would be invaluable. In particular, advice from health service researchers, statisticians, behavioural psychologists and information technologists would greatly enhance many projects. Access to these experts must however be straightforward and timely. Management has a role to play in developing and resourcing these links at an institutional level.

Finding adequate time to complete projects is one of the most commonly encountered problems. Therefore, formal recognition should be given of the time taken to conduct all stages of the audit process. Unless protected time is set aside for clinicians, and built into contracts and work schedules, then establishing high quality audit as an integral part of professional practice will be severely hampered. The provision of protected time by management could be accompanied by a commitment from staff to produce written reports and evidence that the study findings had been acted upon. Balancing this with the need for confidentiality will require care.

Money, even in relatively small amounts, can buy resources in support of audit and can send a strong signal that such activity is valued. Thus funding can act as both a motivator and a facilitator. Within many NHS organizations there is a lack of knowledge of the procedures for disbursing audit funds and some discontent with the process of doing so. To overcome the view that some staff groups have preferential access to funds, greater efforts should be made to describe clearly the process of application. This process should also be streamlined to make it not just fair but also expeditious.

Difficulties surrounding the dynamics of audit groups suggest that multidisciplinary audit activities are not always practical or useful for clinicians. In addition, the conduct of multidisciplinary audit may in itself appear threatening. Thus unidisciplinary audits should also be recognized as legitimate and valuable projects which can contribute to improved quality. Funding arrangements and other institutional support should reflect this. At the same time action is needed to overcome the difficulties posed by multidisciplinary ventures. In part this will be achieved by fostering a supportive climate for audit but it may also need staff training in interpersonal skills in dealing with cross-boundary conflict.

Finally, practical solutions such as the mechanization of routine data collection and computerized notekeeping have been found to both encourage and improve audit activity amongst clinicians. Yet, clinicians often report that data collection is the most demanding part of conducting audit because of the time involved and the tediousness of the task. Greater access to information technology support and the introduction of systems which do away with the necessity of the manual trawling of patients' notes would facilitate the downloading of data and reduce the inappropriate use of staff's clinical time.

Concluding Remarks

The lack of audit expertise among clinicians, and poor institutional responses to the difficulties encountered, have led to haphazard audit activity on a wide scale. Studies of audit programmes have shown that their organization varies widely between hospitals and that most projects fail to adhere to a common goal or purpose (Walshe, 1995; Buttery et al., 1994, 1995a). Consequently many audits rely on a few enthusiasts to keep them going (Kerrison et al., 1993) – but even the enthusiasts lack good audit tools (Gabbay et al,. 1990; Millard, 1996). Access to resources and advice remains a major problem.

The practical and attitudinal barriers to undertaking audit are clearly restraining its progress. Many projects fail to meet their objectives, get scaled-back, or are even abandoned. Few produce clear and demonstrable gains in patient care (although they may produce a wide range of other valued by-products). Consequently audit is not high on the daily agenda of many clinicians, who are often struggling to cope with the increasing demands of their clinical workload. It seems apparent that unless the barriers to successful audit are diminished, and audit activity is both facilitated and valued by managers and peers, then it will fail to become an effective and integral part of clinical care.

Evaluations of audit programmes have shown that providing funding for audit without a well-defined audit programme and support from a skilled and proactive audit department does not necessarily lead to successful audit projects. Evaluation of re-engineered audit programmes needs to continue to ensure the most effective targeting of resources and to identify opportunities for improvement (Barton et al., 1995; Buxton, 1994). In addition, strategies to resolve the barriers confronting clinicians need to be put in place by management. Such evidence of a tangible commitment to audit by managers might help to convince those clinicians who are still ambivalent about the value of audit. Conversely, a lack of commitment from management will ultimately dissuade those who are enthusiastic from continuing their current activity, and will further alienate the sceptics.

Quality improvement remains firmly at the centre of the government's new agenda for the National Health Service. Clinical audit can play an important role in making that concept a reality. Disillusionment with progress to date reflects the superficial and inadequate design of many existing audit programmes. Before we dismiss audit as ineffectual *per se*, much more could be done to ensure that coherent programmes are put in place which are mindful of known problems and are appropriately resourced. Unless significant advances are made in this direction then the claims made for confidential profession-led self-examination will crumble under scrutiny. It then seems likely that public and externally-driven modes of quality assurance will rise in their stead (Davies, 1997; Davies and Lampel, 1998).

Notes

1   For reasons of brevity, the term 'clinicians' will be used throughout the chapter to mean 'health care professionals', i.e. all those with direct care duties including doctors, nurses and the various professions allied to medicine.
2   This and the other quotes throughout the chapter were gathered during a national study of audit in Scotland carried out by the authors (Johnston et al., 1998).

References

Baker, R., Robertson, N. and Farooqi, A. (1995), 'Audit in general practice: factors influencing participation', *British Medical Journal*, 311, pp. 31–4.

Barton, A. and Spencer, J. (1994), 'Differences in attitudes towards audit among specialties in the Northern Region', *Medical Audit News*, 4 (5), pp. 78–9.

Barton, A., Thomson, R. and Bhopal, R. (1995), 'Clinical audit: more research is required', *Journal of Epidemiology and Community Health*, 49, pp. 445–7.

Bennett, J. and Coles, J. (1996), *Evaluating audit. Brighton Health Care NHS Trust's clinical audit programme. A case study*, Caspe Research, London.

Berger, A. (1998), 'Why doesn't audit work?', editorial, *British Medical Journal*, 316, pp. 875–6.

Black, N. (1998), 'Clinical Governance: fine words or action?', *British Medical Journal*, 326, pp. 297–8.

Black, N. and Thompson, E. (1993), 'Obstacles to medical audit: British doctors speak', *Social Science and Medicine*, 36 (7), pp. 849–56.

Buttery, Y., Rumsey, M., Bennett, J. and Coles, J. (1995b), *Evaluating audit. Dorset Healthcare NHS Trust's clinical audit programme. A case study*, Caspe Research, London.

Buttery, Y., Walshe, K., Coles, J. and Bennett, J. (1994), *The development of audit. Findings of a national survey of healthcare provider units in England*, Caspe Research, London.

Buttery, Y., Walshe, K., Rumsey, M., Amess, M., Bennett, J. and Coles, J. (1995a), *Evaluating audit. Provider audit in England. A review of twenty-nine programmes*, Caspe Research, London.

Buxton, M.J. (1994), 'Achievements of audit in the NHS', *Quality in Health Care*, 3, Supplement, s31–4.

Chambers, R., Bowyer, S. and Campbell, I. (1995), 'Audit activity and quality of completed audit projects in primary care in Staffordshire', *Quality in Health Care*, 4, pp. 178–83.

Cooper, A. and French, D. (1993), 'Illustrative examples of successful audit in General Practice', *Audit Trends*, 1, pp. 166–9.

Crombie, I.K and Davies, H.T.O. (1992), 'Towards good audit', *British Journal of Hospital Medicine*, 48, pp. 182–5.

Crombie, I.K and Davies, H.T.O. (1994), 'What is successful audit?', *Managing Audit in General Practice*, 2, pp. 6–8.

Crombie, I.K., Davies, H.T.O., Abraham, S.C.S. and Florey, C. du V. (1993), *The Audit Handbook: Improving Health Care through Clinical Audit*, John Wiley & Sons, Chichester.

Davies, C., Fletcher, J., Wilmot, J. and Szczepura, A. (1995), 'Co-ordinated audit in Warwickshire 1991-1993', *Audit Trends*, 3, pp. 121–6.

Davies, H.T.O. (1997), 'What's a healthy outcome?', *Health Service Journal*, 107 (5548), p. 22.

Davies, H.T.O. and Lampel, J. (1998), 'Trust in Performance Indicators', *Quality in Health Care*, 7, pp. 159–62.

Davies, H.T.O. and Mannion, R. (1999), 'Clinical governance: striking a balance between checking and trusting' in P.C. Smith (ed.), *Reforming markets in health care – an economic perspective*, Open University Press, Milton Keynes.

Davison, K. and Smith, L. (1993), 'Time spent by doctors on medical audit', *Psychiatric Bulletin*, 17, pp. 418–19.

Department of Health (1989), *Working for patients*, HMSO, London.

Department of Health (1997), *Designed to Care. Renewing the National Health Service in Scotland*, The Stationery Office, Edinburgh.

Eccles, M.P., Deverill, M., McColl, E. and Richardson, H. (1996), 'A national survey of audit activity across the primary-secondary care interface', *Quality in Health Care*, 5, pp. 193–200.

Eccles, M.P., Hunt, J. and Newton, J. (1995), 'A case study of an interface audit group', *Audit Trends*, 3, pp. 127–31.

Farrell, L. (1995), 'Audit my shorts', *British Medical Journal*, 311, p. 1171.

Firth-Cozens, J. and Storer, D. (1992), 'Registrars' and senior registrars' perceptions of their audit activities', *Quality in Health Care*, 1, pp. 161–4.

Foster, J., Willmot, M. and Coles, J. (1996), *Evaluating audit. Nursing and therapy audit. An evaluation of twenty four projects and initiatives*, Caspe Research, London.

Fulton, R.A. (1996), 'Goals and methods of audit should be reappraised', *British Medical Journal*, 312, p. 1103.

Gabbay, J. and Layton, A.J. (1992), 'Evaluation of audit of medical inpatient records in a district general hospital', *Quality in Health Care*, 1, pp. 43–7.

Gabbay, J., McNicol, M.C., Spiby, J., Davies, S.C. and Layton, A.J. (1990), 'What did audit achieve? Lessons from preliminary evaluation of a year's medical audit', *British Medical Journal*, 301, pp. 526–9.

Greenhalgh, T. (1992), 'Audit', *British Medical Journal*, 305, p. 961.

Grol, R. and Wensing, M. (1995), 'Implementation of quality assurance and medical audit: general practitioners' perceived obstacles and requirements', *British Journal of General Practice*, 45, pp. 548–52.

Hearnshaw, H.M., Baker, R.H. and Robertson, N. (1994), 'Multidisciplinary audit in primary health care teams: facilitation by audit support staff', *Quality in Health Care*, 3, pp. 164–8.

Hopkins, A. (1996), 'Clinical audit: time for a reappraisal?', *Journal of the Royal College of Physicians of London*, 30 (5), pp. 415–25.

Johnson, R. (1994), 'Where have all the pennies gone? The work of Manchester medical audit advisory group', *British Medical Journal*, 309, pp. 98–102.

Johnston, G., Crombie, I.K., Davies, H.T.O., Alder, E.M. and Millard, A. (1998), 'Barriers to successful audit: what are they and how can they be overcome?', report, Clinical Resource and Audit Group, The Scottish Office, Edinburgh.

Karran, S.J., Ranaboldo, C.J. and Karran, A. (1993), 'Review of the perceptions of general surgical staff within the Wessex region of the status of quality assurance and surgical audit', *Annals of the Royal College of Surgeons of England*, 75, Supplement, pp. 104–7.

Kerrison, S., Packwood, T. and Buxton, M. (1993), *Medical audit. Taking stock*, King's Fund Centre, London.

Kinn, S.R. and Smith, P.J. (1996), 'Medical audit activity in primary and secondary care in the West of Scotland', *Health Bulletin*, 54 (3), pp. 252–7.

Lervy, B., Wareham, K. and Cheung, W.Y. (1994), 'Practice characteristics associated with audit activity: a medical audit advisory group survey', *British Journal of General Practice*, 44 (384), pp. 311–14.

Lewis, C. and Combes, D. (1996), 'Is general practice audit alive and well? The view from Portsmouth', *British Journal of General Practice*, 46, pp. 735–6.

Lord, J. and Littlejohns, P. (1994), 'Secret Garden', *Health Service Journal*, 104 (5417), pp. 18–20.

Lough, J.R.M., McKay, J. and Murray, T.S. (1995a), 'Audit and summative assessment: two years' pilot experience', *Medical Education*, 29, pp. 101–3.

Lough, J.R.M., McKay, J. and Murray, T.S. (1995b), 'Audit: trainers' and trainees' attitudes and experiences', *Medical Education*, 29, pp. 85–90.

Maynard, A. (1991), 'Case for auditing audit', *Health Service Journal*, 101 (5261), p. 26.

McKenna, H.P. (1995), 'A multiprofessional approach to audit', *Nursing Standard*, 9 (46), pp. 32–5.

Miles, A., Bentley, P., Polychronis, A., Price, N. and Grey, J. (1996), 'Clinical audit in the National Health Service: fact or fiction?', *Journal of Evaluation in Clinical Practice*, 2 (1), pp. 29–35.

Millard, A. (1996), 'Health professionals' needs: audit reports', *Audit Trends*, 4, pp. 129–32.

Mooney, G. and Ryan, M. (1992), 'Rethinking medical audit: the goal is efficiency', *Journal of Epidemiology and Community Health*, 46, pp. 180–3.

National Audit Office (1994), *Auditing Clinical Care in Scotland*, HMSO, London.

Nolan, M. and Scott, G. (1993), 'Audit: an exploration of some tensions and paradoxical expectations', *Journal of Advanced Nursing*, 18, pp. 759–66.

Penney, G.C. and Templeton, A. (1995), 'Impact of a national audit project on gynaecologists in Scotland', *Quality in Health Care*, 4, pp. 37–9.

Pringle, M., Bradley, C., Carmichael, C., Wallis, H. and Moore, A. (1994), 'A survey of attitudes to and experience of medical audit in General Practice: Implications for MAAGS', *Audit Trends*, 2, pp. 9–13.

Robinson, S. (1996a), 'Audit in the therapy professions: some constraints on progress', *Quality in Health Care*, 5, pp. 206–14.

Robinson, S. (1996b), 'Evaluating the progress of clinical audit', *The International Journal of Theory, Research and Practice*, 2 (4), pp. 373–92.

Rumsey, M., Buttery, Y., Bennett, J. and Coles, J. (1996a), *Evaluating audit. North Staffordshire's joint clinical audit programme*, Caspe Research, London.

Rumsey, M., Buttery, Y., Bennett, J. and Coles, J. (1996b), *Wythenshawe Hospital's clinical audit programme. A case study*, CASPE Research, London.

Secretary of State for Health (1998), *A First Class Service: Quality in the New NHS*, Department of Health, London.

Sellu, D. (1996), 'Time to audit audit', *British Medical Journal*, 312, pp. 128–9.

Sherwood, T. (1992), 'Exitus auditus – no fun', *The Lancet*, 340, pp. 37–8.

Smith, H.E., Russell, G.I., Frew, A.J. and Dawes, P.T. (1992), 'Medical audit: the differing perspectives of managers and clinicians', *Journal of the Royal College of Physicians of London*, 26 (2), pp. 177–80.

Spencer, J.A. (1992), 'Audit and academic departments of general practice: a survey in the United Kingdom and Eire', *British Journal of General Practice*, 42, pp. 333–5.

Tabandeh, H. and Thompson, G.M. (1995), 'Auditing ophthalmology audits', *Eye*, 9, Supplement, pp. 1–5.

Thomson, R.G. and Barton, A.G. (1994), 'Is audit running out of steam?', *Quality in Health Care*, 3, pp. 225–9.

Thomson, R.G., Elcoat, C. and Pugh, G. (1996), 'Clinical audit and the purchaser-provider interaction: different attitudes and expectations in the United Kingdom', *Quality in Health Care*, 5, pp. 97–103.

Toy, P.T.C.Y. (1994), 'Effectiveness of transfusion audits and practice guidelines', *Archives of Pathology Laboratory Medicine*, 118, pp. 435–7.

Walshe, K. (1995), 'The traits of success in clinical audit' in K. Walshe (ed.), *Evaluating clinical audit; past lessons, future directions*, conference proceedings, The Royal Society of Medicine Press, London.

Walshe, K. and Coles, J. (1995), 'Introduction' in K. Walshe (ed.), *Evaluating clinical audit; past lessons, future directions*, conference proceedings, The Royal Society of Medicine Press, London.

Watkins, C.J. and King, J. (1996), 'Understanding the barriers to medical audit: insights from the experience of one practice', *Audit Trends*, 4, pp. 47–52.

Webb, M.D. and Harvey, I.M. (1992), 'Taking stock of medical audit: a questionnaire survey', *Medical Audit News*, 2 (2), p. 18.

Webb, M.D. and Harvey, I.M. (1994), 'Auditing the introduction of audit', *Medical Audit News*, 4 (2), pp. 19–20.

Webb, S.J., Dowell, A.C. and Heywood, P. (1991), 'Survey of general practice audit in Leeds', *British Medical Journal*, 302, pp. 390–2.

Willmot, M., Foster, J., Walshe, K. and Coles, J. (1995), *A review of audit activity in the nursing and therapy professions. Findings of a national survey*, Caspe Research, London.

7 Improving Child Dental Health in Scotland: An Audit in Primary Care

CHRIS SOUTHWICK,[1] DAFYDD EVANS[2] AND HUW T.O. DAVIES[3]

1   *General Dental Practitioner*
2   *Dundee Dental School*
3   *Department of Management, University of St Andrews*

Introduction

Dental disease is a major public health problem in the UK. Nearly a quarter of adults have no natural teeth of their own, and of those adults who do have teeth, nine out of 10 have amalgam fillings (Todd and Lader, 1988). Children's dental health is just as poor, with 62 per cent of all Scottish five year-olds having some decayed teeth (Pitts and Palmer, 1995). The cost of meeting this health need is considerable. In Scotland, over 90 per cent of all primary dental care is provided by around 1,800 general dental practitioners (GDPs) working in independent practice. In 1996/97 GDPs provided treatment to the value of £140 million for Scotland's population of five million people (SDPB, 1997). Of this figure, 15 per cent was spent preventing and managing dental decay in children. Is this expenditure on child dental health managing effectively the problem of dental disease in children? The available evidence indicates that it is not.

Despite 95 per cent of Scottish five year-olds having been taken to see a dentist at least once (O'Brien, 1994), only about 10 per cent of dental decay in five year-olds' teeth is treated (Pitts and Palmer, 1995). Untreated dental decay in children usually leads to extractions, and by the time they reach eight years of age, 42 per cent of Scottish children will have had at least one tooth extracted (O'Brien, 1994). Extractions can usually be avoided by advanced dental procedures such as root fillings and stainless steel crowns,

Managing Quality: Strategic Issues in Health Care Management, H.T.O. Davies, M. Tavakoli, M. Malek, A.R. Neilson (eds), Ashgate Publishing Ltd, 1999.

but these are rarely used. For example, in 1996/97 121,000 teeth were extracted from children, the great majority because of decay, yet in a seven month period within that year for which data were available, only 2,500 baby teeth were root treated, and only 154 stainless steel crowns were fitted (SDPB, 1997). Why is so much dental decay in children receiving inadequate treatment, despite free and widespread access to dental care?

General dental practitioners work as independent contractors within the National Health Service. For many years there has been no tradition of a quality assessment infrastructure within their workplace. The Scottish Dental Practice Board, who authorize Health Boards to pay GDPs on behalf of the Secretary of State, can arrange for patients who have completed a course of treatment with a GDP to be screened by the Regional Dental Officer service. However, the average GDP can expect to have only three or four patients a year screened, and it is unlikely that this figure will include more than one child. In general, then, GDPs are the sole arbiters of the quality of treatment provided within their own practice, yet it is uncertain whether they have the skills and motivation to carry out this assessment effectively. In recent years, this lack of support for quality assessment in practice has been recognized, with the appointment in each region of a GDP Audit Facilitator, to encourage GDPs to conduct audit projects within their practices. Nevertheless, the precise reasons for the inadequacies in child dental care in practice remain uncertain. Anecdotal evidence from GDPs indicates that a variety of factors might be involved. These include poorly motivated patients and parents, poor morale amongst GDPs, inadequate fees and lack of knowledge about best practice. However, there is a lack of data in this area and it was this deficiency that the present study set out to address.

Aims

The aim of this project was twofold. Firstly, to determine factors contributing to the poor quality of child dental care in Scotland. Second, to assess the feasibility of involving GDPs in the development of evidence-based guidelines for successful application in primary care. More specifically, the study aimed to:

- determine what dentists currently do for their child patients;
- assess what dentists think they ought to be doing;
- establish agreed evidence-based guidelines (audit standards) for dentists

to implement in order to improve the management and prevention of dental decay;
- ensure professional ownership of these standards by local GDPs;
- disseminate these audit standards;
- reassess the clinical practice in children's dentistry;
- assess the changes achieved, identify discrepancies, and determine reasons for those discrepancies;
- identify barriers to change and possible solutions to those barriers.

This chapter reports on the first five of these key aims. In particular, it focuses on the novel attempts to bring GDPs (despite their independent contractor status) into a quality improvement programme.

Method

Developing Audit Standards

The components of a preventive approach to child primary dental care chosen to be included within the audit were:

1 reliable diagnosis of disease including the targeted use of radiographs, which would allow identification of 'high caries risk' children, leading to;

2 appropriate targeting of these children with preventive measures, namely:
  - fissure sealants
  - dentists' advice on fluoride regimes, diet and toothbrushing;

3 together with appropriate restorative management of the decayed teeth.

In order to implement an audit of children's dentistry, audit standards had to be developed as a first stage. These audit standards were based on the evidence-based clinical guidelines 'Targeted Prevention of Dental Caries in the Permanent Dentition of 6–16 year olds presenting for Dental Care', currently being developed by the Scottish Inter-collegiate Guidelines Network (SIGN). In consideration of the above, specific audit standards were derived for the following clinical areas:

- caries diagnosis (use of X-rays);

- fissure sealants;
- dentists' advice on fluoride regimes, diet and toothbrushing;
- restorative management of dental caries.

The first part of the study was to establish current practice with regard to these clinical areas. Following this, GDPs involved in the study were to be invited to attend a meeting at which national guidelines covering these clinical areas (the SIGN guidelines) were to be outlined and their suitability for general dental practice discussed. This would allow modification of the guidelines to suit local requirements and ensure local ownership. The guidelines would then be tested for applicability in general dental practice by a second round of the study, with the same design. The study would then finish with a final meeting to see if a change in clinical practice had occurred and, if not, to determine the barriers to change.

Recruitment of GDPs

Successful audit projects involve not only the recruitment of participants but also the maintenance of their commitment for the duration of the project. Other workers have experienced considerable difficulties in maintaining the cooperation of GDPs in research and audit projects (Mackie, 1998; Joshi and Bhattie, 1998). As this has not been our experience with the current initiative (Evans et al., 1998), the approach to recruitment used will be described in some detail.

General dental practitioners in Tayside, Fife and Grampian were circulated and asked if they might be interested in being involved with research into primary dental care of children. From 121 GDPs contacted in Tayside, there were 110 positive responses. There was a similarly high response rate from Fife (70 positive responses) and Grampian (96 positive responses). From these respondents, a local coordinator was recruited from each of the Health Board regions. Each coordinator was then required to recruit 25 GDPs from the respondents in their region, and to encourage and maintain enthusiasm amongst their GDPs for the duration of the study. The Tayside coordinator (CS) was also the coordinator of the whole project. The dentists were selected to ensure that there was a proportional mix of urban town/city to rural/small town practice locations, year of graduation and males to females.

Dentists initially chosen for inclusion in the study were contacted briefly by telephone to ask them if they would consider taking part in the study programme. The telephone contact to dentists involved:

1 a reminder of their expressed interest in the management of caries in children;

2 a request for a meeting with them to explain a new project for their consideration and involvement.

The project was not described in terms of an audit of individual practitioner care; rather the benefits to practitioners in terms of improved practice were emphasized. This was deliberate as it was considered vital to obtain as accurate a picture as possible of current practice in child dental care, and the mention of an audit could have resulted in a modification of their normal routine practice procedures. At all times in contacts with the GDPs great respect and consideration were given to their time management, and every effort was made for minimal interference with their routine surgery schedules. This was considered not only courteous but also essential by the coordinators who were fully aware of the stresses of interruptions during practice hours. It was also realized that the data collection was going to involve considerable activity and application by the dental team and it was important to maintain good will. Only four of the selected practitioners rejected the request for a meeting to consider the study.

Assessing Current Practice in Children's Dentistry

The first phase of the audit cycle involved finding out 'What dentists do now' in caring for their child patients. In order to assess the current practice, data were collected by each of the 75 dentists in the study on 30 of their child patients (see Table 7.1).

Table 7.1   Age range and number of patients assessed by each general dental practitioner

Age of patients	Number per GDP	Stage of dental development
3–5 years	10	Primary dentition
6–12 years	10	Mixed dentition
13–16 years	10	Permanent dentition

Thus the aim was to collect detailed information on a total of 2,250 children. The sample sizes were chosen to permit significant comparisons to be made within and across Health Board areas. An appropriate clinical data collection sheet was designed, including details of the patient's name and age, the date of the current visit and previous visits, and the dates of previous X-rays together with the reason that they were taken. The patient record sheet had a tear-off copy to enable the dentists to keep the copy in their records to avoid duplication of effort. The data collection sheets were piloted on three GDPs not involved in the study, and modifications were made until completion difficulties were eliminated.

In addition to the details from the record sheets it was decided to supplement the information with a structured questionnaire with each dentist in order to elicit treatment/diagnostic practices covering the areas of audit concern. Questions were designed to determine the quality of clinical care and preventive strategy utilization. All of the questions were designed as 'the closed question' variety but with options and choices in certain areas. The questionnaire was piloted by five GDPs not involved in the study.

Once the protocol for the patient survey was finalized a meeting was arranged with each of the dentists, in order to give them a full explanation of the study and commitment required. The GDPs were individually visited at their surgeries at their convenience. Many were visited over the lunch period or at the end of evening surgery. Several were visited at home at times convenient to their personal circumstances. Every effort was made by the coordinators to minimize disruption to their work or private lives.

Dentists were asked to participate in the initiative by:

1 recording the examination, diagnosis, treatment plan and actual treatment provided to 30 children;

2 completing the detailed questionnaire at a structured face-to-face interview to be conducted after the completion of the patient survey;

3 attending a meeting to consider the results of the patient/dentist data and agree a set of protocols (audit standards) for implementation on another 30 patients;

4 completing another survey of 30 patients after implementing the protocols;

5 attending a final dissemination/discussion meeting to consider effectiveness of implementation of the audit guidelines.

The second phase of the audit cycle, involving reviewing the treatment of another 30 patients, was discussed with each dentist on the basis that the protocols (guidelines) were being introduced to test the ability of a group of dentists to work together to protocols in order to provide standardized procedures for examining the effectiveness of new treatment regimes. The final draft version of the new SIGN guidelines was available in time for the first meeting, and the dentists were happy to test-implement their modifications of these as the basis for the second audit cycle. In this way, the dentists felt as though they were testing somebody else's guidelines and not being 'examined' on their own work.

After explaining the study, the commitment and the procedures the dentists were invited to participate. They were given the choice of informing the study coordinators at that visit, or of contacting them within 10 days with their answer. All dentists who received a personal visit and direct explanation agreed to participate in the project.

Conducting the Patient Survey and Dentist Questionnaires

Each participating dentist received a pack with the protocol; the patient record forms for data collection; a sample charting; an easy check list for recording numbers of patients seen at each age and a covering letter outlining the overall programme commitment. On completion of the treatment on the first five patients, the data sheets were returned in a prepaid envelope for evaluating the standard of recordings. Appropriate contact was made with each dentist by way of encouragement, clarification or correction as necessary. Only a few small administrative or charting errors occurred.

Each dentist was then contacted to arrange a personal visit for completion of the structured questionnaires. The questionnaire required an average of 25 minutes for completion. Each dentist was given a questionnaire and asked to give his/her answers to the interviewer who was present only to ensure adequate understanding of the questions and not for prompting in any way. A standardized format of approach was agreed and adopted by the coordinators in conducting these questionnaires.

Results

Best Practice, Stated Practice and Actual Practice

The dentists provided treatment schedules and examinations of 2,005 children.

Analysis of the data from these patients indicated that they were a representative cross-section of patients from the Health Board areas in terms of the number under regular dental care, males to females and decay experience. An analysis of the treatment regimes and prevention strategies from the patient forms provided a clear pattern of current treatment practices. A direct comparison could also be made with the dentists' statements about intended practice as recorded on the dentist questionnaires.

Utilization of X-rays for Caries Diagnosis

The audit standard is that all children should have X-rays at least every two years from the age of five years until 18 years of age, in order to allow early detection of dental caries and its appropriate management (SIGN, 1998). Analysis was made of the patient records to determine the utilization of X-rays in caries diagnosis over the previous 24 months. The actual use on patients was then compared with the dentists responses to the questionnaires on X-ray utilization. Dentists' statements about utilizing X-rays fell short of the SIGN guidelines recommendations, and in practice, few children actually received X-rays (see Table 7.2).

Table 7.2   Dentists reported X-ray utilization and their actual utilization

Age band of patients (years)	Recommended utilization of X-rays (%)	Dentists stating they would X-ray (%)	Patients actually receiving X-rays (%)
6–12	100	50.0	5.1
13–16	100	91.5	19.3

Preventive measures

Preventive measures include:

- fissure sealing;
- advice from the dentist on fluoride regimes, diet and toothbrushing.

With regard to fissure sealing, over half of the decay occurring in molar teeth starts in the deep fissures on the surface of the tooth, and can be prevented by flowing a thin layer of plastic resin over the fissures. This is a simple procedure, and the audit standards are clear that all first and second molars should be sealed if children have one or more carious teeth (SIGN, 1998). When the dentists were asked in the questionnaire how consistently they sealed first and second molars, 58 per cent of dentists always or usually sealed all the first molars and 30 per cent always or usually sealed the second molars. Analysis of the patient records, however, showed that 40 per cent of the children had their first molars sealed and 22 per cent had their second molars sealed, and that there was no difference between those who were caries-free and those who had one or more decayed teeth. This indicates that some dentists are sealing all the children's molars irrespective of decay level (risk category) whilst others are sealing none.

The questionnaires indicated that 91 per cent of dentists said that they routinely gave their patients advice about the use of fluoride toothpaste, 49 per cent said they routinely gave diet advice and 83 per cent said they routinely gave toothbrushing instruction. However, the patient returns indicated advice being given considerably less often than this (Table 7.3).

Table 7.3   Patients actually given oral health advice

Age band of patients (years)	Diet advice	Fluoride advice	Toothbrush instruction
6–12	8.6%	1.5%	5.3%
13–16	7.4%	1.8%	8.1%

Management of Dental Caries

When examining the number of children who had their primary molar teeth restored as a percentage of the number of children with decay, it was found that 69 per cent of the children had their carious teeth restored. For five year-old children this was 70 per cent. This is a higher proportion than was found in previous surveys (Pitts and Palmer, 1995).

Current Dental Practice in Summary

Although the proportion of decayed baby teeth being filled was higher than expected, for all measures there was a big gap between best practice, stated practice and actual practice. The reasons for this are unclear at this stage of the audit, but there are indications that there may be a financial basis. When asked to list in order of priority the factors they considered most important in improving the quality of child dental care, three of the top four items were related to having more time to spend with the patient on matters such as diet advice and toothbrushing instruction. In fact, 84 per cent of GDPs questioned stated that inadequate resource was a major barrier to providing more effective child dental health care.

Gaining Acceptance and Ownership of Best Practice Standards

The next major task was to derive specific locally agreed audit standards for each of the clinical areas of audit. These audit standards had to be practical, clinically acceptable and workable in the NHS practice environment. Ideally they needed to be evidence-based guidelines which could be locally modified for this initiative. Fortunately the Scottish Inter-collegiate Guidelines Network (SIGN) had commissioned a development group, under the chairmanship of Professor Nigel Pitts, to develop evidence-based guidelines for the prevention of dental caries in the permanent teeth of 6–16 year-old children presenting for dental care in Scotland. The SIGN group permitted the use of the draft formulation of the guidelines as a basis for the protocols for this audit project.

Dentists' Meetings – Development of Local Guidelines

The participating dentists in each of the three regions were invited to an evening meeting in their region with the provision of a buffet supper prior to the meeting. This meeting had been an accepted part of the study programme from the start and 42 dentists out of the remaining 70 in the programme attended the meetings, a 60 per cent attendance. The meetings were held on successive evenings in Dundee, Aberdeen and Glenrothes.

These meetings followed the same protocol and enabled a thorough discussion of the proposed guidelines. The GDPs were presented with a summary of the results of the patient survey and the dentist questionnaires. An outline of the philosophy behind the SIGN guidelines was given, followed by a detailed description of the proposed appropriate modification of the guideline for each of the clinical areas of audit. The dentists were then divided into three focus groups in order to discuss two of the guideline areas together with the assessment of caries risk. These discussion groups were thorough and probing, with the dentists providing practical insights into the modification and application of the guidelines. In particular the dentists provided critical and corrective comments on the clinical practicality and economic viability of the guidelines involving these clinical procedures:

1 utilization of X-rays;
2 use of composite sealant restorations;
3 establishing of criteria for caries risk;
4 use of fissure sealants.

Some parts of the guidelines were subject to local modification and others (particularly on diet advice) were given greater clarity. The comments and modifications from the three meetings were assessed and combined to produce an 'agreed' modification to the draft SIGN guidelines. Indeed, the feedback from these meetings enabled the SIGN team themselves to modify their own guidelines in the light of comments and discussion arising from this project.

These guidelines were then structured, simplified, put in colour and laminated for easy use in the surgery. They thus provided an appropriate *aide-memoire* for every day use. A protocol for application of the guidelines was produced and provided to each practitioner together with another charting guide and checklist for recording the patients surveyed.

Each of the practitioners who had not been able to attend the meetings was personally visited, a briefing was given covering the meetings and the conclusions drawn. The philosophy and modifications of the guidelines were also carefully discussed. This enabled all the dentists to identify with and take ownership of the guidelines. The dentists greatly appreciated being informed of the progress of the project and their interest for the second phase of the patient surveys was encouraged and motivated.

In this way specific locally-derived clinical audit standards were disseminated to the GDPs in a practical, easy-to-use format. These protocols had been developed from existing evidence-based guidelines with modifications decided by the actual practitioners participating in the project. It must be noted that considerable commitment was being shown by the practitioners in their acceptance of, and continued involvement in the project. The fact that 70 out of the original 75 GDPs are still involved in the project is remarkable and very encouraging. Further data collection is now ongoing, which will help to determine the effectiveness of this approach in bringing about important changes in practitioner treatment behaviour.

Concluding Remarks

Although the audit project is still ongoing, it is already clear that the project has been successful in securing continued commitment and enthusiasm from GDPs to examine their clinical practice. The drop-out rate amongst the GDPs has been lower than expected, and the quality of the data obtained was higher than anticipated. Discussion with the GDPs has indicated that the following factors were important in this:

- the topic was of interest to the clinicians involved;
- the coordinators were all practising GDPs, fully aware of the difficulties involved in running the project in dental practice;
- the GDPs were all fully informed of the commitment required prior to recruitment;
- all the data collection sheets and questionnaires were extensively piloted with GDPs prior to the start of the study;
- through the group meetings, all the GDPs felt involved in the study, rather than just passive participants;
- the three coordinators were all highly motivated.

So far, the most important finding of the study is that, at present, dental treatment for children falls far short of the levels set by the evidence-based audit standards, while the most interesting finding is that there is sometimes a large discrepancy between what practitioners know they ought to do and what they actually do. This study shows that it is possible to run successful audit projects in primary care (even with independent contractors), but that considerable preparation and commitment is required to achieve committed participation.[1]

Note

1   This work was funded by the Clinical Resource and Audit Group (CRAG) of the Scottish Office. We are very grateful to CRAG for this funding. Nonetheless, the views expressed in this paper are those of the authors and do not necessarily reflect those of either CRAG or The Scottish Office.

References

Evans, D.J.P., Southwick, C.A.P. and Davies, H.T.O. (1998), 'Clinical Trials in Primary Dental Care', *British Dental Journal*, 185, pp. 110–1.

Joshi, R.I. and Bhatti, S.A. (1998), 'Research Problems in Primary Care', *British Dental Journal* 184, p. 470.

Mackie, I.C. (1998), 'Evidence-based Research in the Primary Dental Care Setting', *British Dental Journal* 184, p. 6.

O'Brien, M. (1994), *Childrens' Dental Health in the United Kingdom 1993*, OPCS, HMSO, London.

Pitts, N.B. and Palmer, J.D. (1995), 'The Dental Caries Experience of 5-year-old Children in Great Britain. Surveys Co-ordinated by the British Association for the Study of Community Dentistry in 1993/94', *Community Dental Health*, 12, pp. 52–8.

Scottish Dental Practice Board Annual Report 1996/97, Trinity Park House, Edinburgh.

Scottish Inter-collegiate Guidelines Network (1998, in preparation), *Targeted Prevention of Dental Caries in the Permanent Dentition of 6–16 year olds presenting for Dental Care*, SIGN Secretariat, Royal College of Physicians, Edinburgh.

Todd, J.E. and Lader,D. (1991), *Adult Dental Health, 1988, UK*, HMSO, London.

8 Human Resource Management Audits: Contributions to Quality

SANDRA NUTLEY
Department of Management, University of St Andrews

Introduction

It is widely recognized that quality is multidimensional (Donabedian, 1980; Maxwell, 1992). This multidimensionality relates both to how we define quality (see Figure 8.1) and to the ways in which organizations can act to improve quality. There are a number of quality assessment frameworks which might provide a guide for organizations seeking continuous improvement in their activities and results. One such generic framework is the European Foundation of Quality Management (EFQM) business excellence model. This model (see Figure 8.2) consists of nine elements which are grouped into two broad areas: enablers – how we do things; results – what we target, measure and achieve. Organizations are encouraged to undertake a comprehensive and systematic review of their activities and results, using the nine elements of the business excellence model. This chapter considers one of the nine elements identified by the EFQM model – people management.

In 1998 Sam Galbraith (Minister for Health, Scotland) launched the Human Resource Strategy for the NHS in Scotland (NHSiS) with the following words:

> the Plan for Managing People is, I believe, a major step forward in helping enable people who work in the NHS in Scotland to continue to deliver high quality patient care as we approach the millennium and beyond (The Scottish Office, 1998, p. v).

It seems a truism to suggest that in health care organizations quality of

Managing Quality: Strategic Issues in Health Care Management, H.T.O. Davies, M. Tavakoli, M. Malek, A.R. Neilson (eds), Ashgate Publishing Ltd, 1999.

Effectiveness – technical quality of treatment
Acceptability – the way in which the service is delivered
Efficiency – maximum output for a given input
Access – availability of treatment when it is needed
Equity – fair treatment of patients relative to others
Relevance – appropriate balance of services given the needs and wants
   of the population as a whole

Figure 8.1   Maxwell's six dimensions of quality

Source: Maxwell, 1992, p. 171.

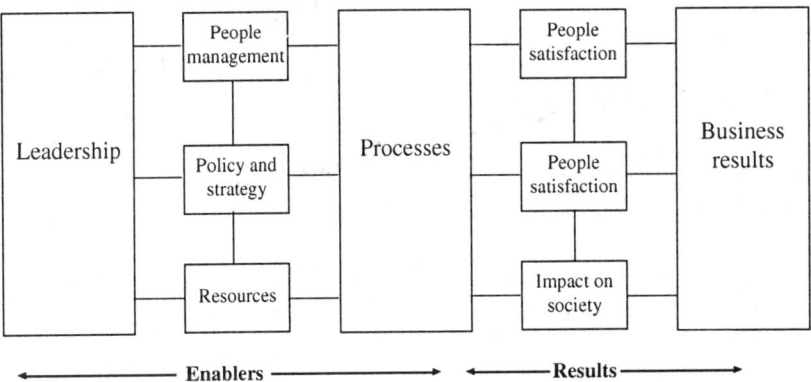

Figure 8.2   EFQM business excellence model

Source: British Quality Foundation, undated, p. 5. Copyright: British Quality
   Foundation and EFQM.

service is highly dependent on the quality of the staff who deliver those
services. Having staff with the right knowledge, skills and commitment is an
important ingredient for improving both the technical quality of a service and
its acceptability to service users. The key issue is how organizations ensure
that they have the right staff in the right place, at the right time and for the
right price. This is the role of human resource management (HRM). An
assessment of the success of HRM in achieving these aims is one of the tasks
of HRM audits.

There is anecdotal evidence that HRM audits are on the increase in public
service organizations. The reasons for the increase are likely to involve a
number of factors. For example, the shift from personnel management to

human resource management (see below) places the implementation of an HR strategy in the hands of line managers and there have been suggestions that their practices may need auditing (McGovern et al., 1997). The increase in HRM audits may also be a reflection of the 'audit explosion' in society more generally (Power, 1994 and 1997). Within the NHS there has been increased interest in evaluating/benchmarking HRM effectiveness. This is in part a response to the scrutiny of management and support services costs in the wake of the 1997 White Papers on NHS. A variety of models for evaluating HRM effectiveness are being considered. For example, in Scotland eight NHS Trusts are participating in a pilot of the Accounts Commission's Managing People audit framework (Accounts Commission, 1997).

This chapter considers the contribution of human resource management (HRM) audits to improving the quality of health care services. In doing so it addresses three main questions:

1   what does an HRM audit entail?;

2   is there any one methodology for auditing HRM which is likely to be more beneficial than other possible approaches?;

3   what do we know about the effectiveness of HRM in the NHS and is there evidence that auditing HRM increases this effectiveness with the desired effect of improving the quality of health care services?

The three main sections of this chapter discuss each of these questions in turn.

Before moving on to consider the various approaches to HRM auditing, it is important to define how the concept of human resource management is used in this chapter. Clarifying what is meant by human resource management and in what ways, if any, this is different to personnel management is a potential minefield. As Storey (1995, p. 4) points out 'HRM as a concept has been, and remains, highly controversial'. The hallmark of HRM for some commentators (e.g. Open Business School, 1992) is the degree to which human resource practices are consistent with each other and integrated with an organization's strategy. It is not appropriate to debate here whether HRM is fundamentally different to personnel management (for this, see Legge, 1989 and 1995): suffice to say that HRM is used in this paper as the generic term rather than personnel management. Where there is a need to refer to the potentially distinctive nature of an HRM doctrine, this is referred to as the HRM ideology. The term personnel is used when wishing to refer explicitly to those staff working in personnel or HR departments.

What Does an HRM Audit Entail?

Defining what an HRM audit is and, conversely, what it is not is fraught with difficulties. Power (1997) argues that there is no precise agreement about what auditing is as compared with other types of evaluative practice, such as inspection or assessment. He does, however, outline a number of generally accepted ingredients of audit practice:

> *independence* from the matter being audited; technical work in the form of *evidence* gathering and the examination of documentation; the expression of a *view* based on the evidence; a clearly defined *object* of the process (Power, 1997, p. 5, original emphasis).

An important ingredient missing from the above characterization of audit practice is any requirement for action in response to audit findings. Clearly if HRM audits are to lead to improvement in the quality of health care services, they need to connect with meaningful action.

Defining the appropriate object of an HRM audit is the subject of debate. Nutley (1998) has developed a typology of HRM audits which suggests that there are at least seven ways in which the scope and objectives of such an audit may be drawn:

* *Scope 1: Compliance Audit*

An assessment of the extent to which organizational practices comply with existing human resource policies and procedures.

* *Scope 2: Systems Audit*

A review of existing human resource policies and procedures to ensure that they provide an internally coherent and strategically relevant management system. Such an audit would compare the existing control system with templates reflecting best practice guidelines.

- *Scope 3: Performance Audit*

  A review of the performance emanating from existing human resource management systems, using indicators such as: turnover rates, stability indices, sickness and absenteeism rates. Such indicators would be compared with a number of yardsticks (e.g. past performance, other organizations and targets or standards) to assess the scope for improving performance.

- *Scope 4: User Satisfaction Audit*

  An audit may look beyond the traditional roles of personnel staff in providing employment services and focus on the broader consultancy role of personnel staff. Such an audit would assess the effectiveness of personnel staff in undertaking this role, and is likely to rely on surveying the satisfaction levels of those using personnel consultancy services.

- *Scope 5: Value-added Audit*

  An evaluation of the value-added by the personnel function – employing techniques such as human asset accounting and cost benefit analysis. Such evaluations aim to compare, for example, the cost of training with a valuation of the benefits of this training.

- *Scope 6: Strategic HRM Audit*

  An appraisal of whether human resources are being managed strategically and whether personnel staff, in particular, play a strategic role. Such an audit is likely to focus on appraising the HR strategy and examining the input of personnel staff into the development of corporate strategies and their role in implementing these strategies.

- *Scope 7: Organization and People Audit*

  An audit which explicitly moves beyond the personnel function and its systems by incorporating a broader consideration of how the organization deploys, manages and utilizes its human resources.

  These categories are not hard and fast or mutually exclusive. Any specific audit may combine two or more of these ways of scoping the audit. Audit scopes 1 and 2, and to some extent scopes 3 and 4, have reasonably well developed frameworks and methodologies. The methodological development of audit scopes 5, 6 and 7 are still very much in their infancy.

It is important not to confuse human resource management audits with an audit of human resources. The former is concerned with assessing the ways in which an organization deploys, manages and utilizes its employees. The latter reflects one of the means an organization might use to assist it with staff planning.

Choosing an Appropriate HRM Audit Approach

The overall aim of an HRM audit should be to affect the way in which people are managed in order to improve overall organizational performance. The question which, therefore, arises is whether any of the above audit approaches are better than others in achieving this aim. The audit approaches can be divided crudely into those which focus on systems/process and those which are concerned with performance (outputs and outcomes). Audits have traditionally been concerned with ensuring that good systems are in place. However, the effect of the HRM ideology has been to shift attention to ends rather than means. Storey (1995, p. 7) points out that the HRM ideology shifts the emphasis away from personnel procedures and rules as the basis of good practice, in favour of a new emphasis on the management of culture. Culture is the preferred control mechanism and performance is the goal. Torrington (1993) argues that this emphasis on performance rather than conformity to rules and formal controls is of value in ensuring that HRM activities are developed within organizations.

Expanding the scope of HRM auditing to include performance review seeks to avoid assuming that there are set means to an end and also endeavours to focus on fitness for purpose. Performance audits may analyse HR outcomes (e.g. turnover and absenteeism) and/or organizational outcomes (e.g. patient satisfaction). This is in line with various models of HRM; for example, Guest (1987) proposes a range of human resource policies which, if pursued, will result in positive HR outcomes. These, in turn, should result in one or more organizational outcomes. A similar set of associations is proposed by the Harvard analytical framework (see Figure 8.3). There is evidence of a shift in emphasis away from auditing HRM processes to auditing outputs and outcomes in the private (Ulrich, 1998) and public sectors (Collins, 1997), and certainly in health care (Davies and Crombie, 1997). There remain questions about

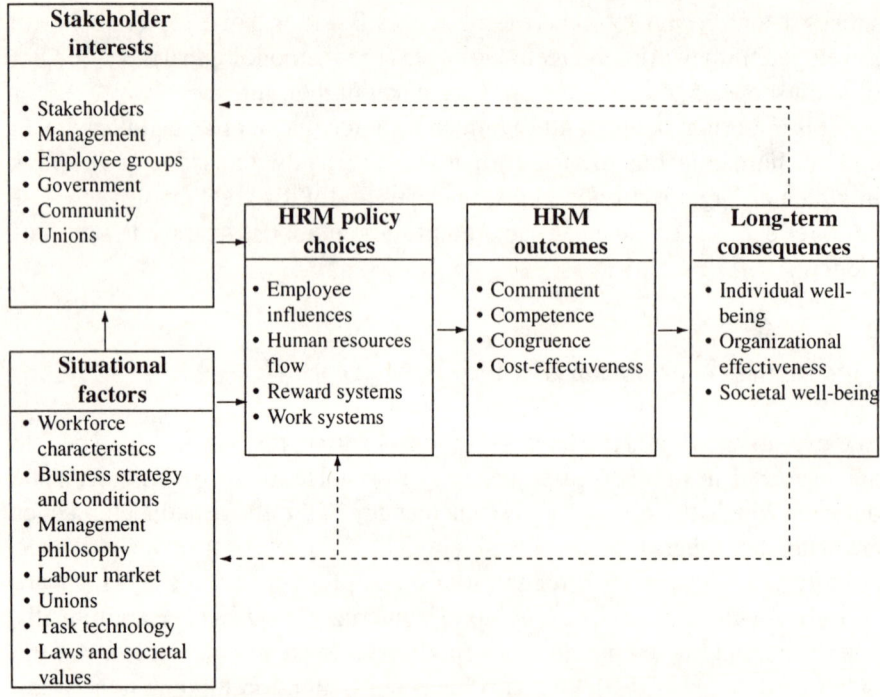

Figure 8.3 The Harvard analytical framework for HRM

Source: Beer et al., 1984, p. 16. Reprinted with the permission of The Free Press, A
        division of Simon and Schuster, Inc. from *Managing Human Assets* by
        Michael Beer, Bert Spector, Paul R. Lawrence, D. Quinn Mills, Richard E.
        Walton. Copyright © 1984 by The Free Press.

how far this is desirable and practical (Davies and Crombie, 1995; Davies,
1998).

HRM systems audits have a number of strengths. Any organization needs
systems to plan, coordinate and control its activities. Information and
communication form the basis of control systems and it is they that make it
possible to run and control a business (Treadway Commission, 1992). As
Power (1997, p. 82) says:

> if one can have confidence that a system exists to control the completeness,
> accuracy and validity of transactions between and organization and its
> environment, then it is unnecessary to duplicate this work and look at transactions
> in detail.

There is no shortage of recommendations about good systems design for HRM. For example, Dolenko (1990) provides a framework which divides the HR function into seven main components: human resources planning, staffing, training, performance appraisals, employee relations, compensation and benefits, and human resource information systems. She then sets out a series of expectations in relation to the systems which should be in place for managing each of these areas. Figure 8.4 illustrates this by setting out the expectations in relation to performance appraisals.

Audit Objective
To determine whether the performance appraisal process assists managers in optimizing the achievement of organisational objectives.

Related Criterion 1: Establishment of Work Expectations
Work expectations should provide terms of reference for the employees with respect to his/her expected contribution to the achievement of organisational objectives.

Related Criterion 2: Ongoing Review and Discussion
There should be ongoing review and discussion of achievement against expectations throughout the review period.

Related Criterion 3: Evaluation of Performance
During an annual review interview, emphasis should be placed on dialogue, mutual problem-solving, recognition of accomplishments, and specific feedback to assist in the improvement of performance.

Related Criterion 4: Monitoring and Evaluation of the Performance Appraisal Process
Monitoring and evaluation of the performance appraisal process should ensure that performance reviews are occurring in accordance with the criteria which have been set by the organisation.

The expected control system for each criterion is further elaborated in the framework. For example, for criterion 3:
a) The annual review should:
•   Reflect the results of ongoing review and discussions.
•   Be constructive in tone in order to assist the employee with self-assessment and/ or improvement.
•   Identify training and development needs (as required).
•   Establish work expectations for the next review period.
b) The review of each employee's performance should be summarised in an appraisal report at least annually.

Figure 8.4   Dolenko's audit framework for performance appraisal

Source: Dolenko, 1990, pp. 18–19.

In a similar vein, the Account Commission (Accounts Commission, 1995) in their review of management processes in NHS trusts in Scotland, proposed a number of good practice components which apply to the personnel function. These include:

- a clearly defined role for the human resources department;
- the establishment of priority objectives;
- clearly defined personnel duties of line managers and the personnel department which are understood by all members of staff;
- the production of a staffing plan to meet the required level of service;
- clearly identifiable costs of running the human resources department and a regular review of these costs and value of service;
- the possession of a trust human resources plan which is linked to its business and corporate plans;
- review of all trust personnel policies by the board;
- a structure in place to keep staff informed of personnel policies and the respective responsibilities of line managers and the personnel department.

The Accounts Commission (1995) report that the majority of NHS trusts they visited had most of this good practice in place.

Clark (1994) argues that the principles of fairness and consistency should be the guide to management action and he is critical of strategic HRM's downgrading of the importance of systems and procedures. The demands of public accountability and fairness, in addition to the need for efficiency and effectiveness, imply that public service organizations cannot afford to ignore operational procedures. Hence systems audits should be of value.

The problem is that good systems do not necessarily equate with good performance and systems audits can provide assurance that the system works well even when substantive performance is poor (Power, 1997). There is a danger that systems audits demonstrate fitness for audit rather than fitness for purpose. The audit literature (Bowerman, 1996; Power, 1997) talks of an 'expectations gap'; more is expected from systems auditing than it can deliver. If this is the case, then systems audits of HRM may provide audit committees with either a false sense of security or cause misplaced concern. A false sense of security would arise if seemingly good systems did not produce good services. Misplaced concern would ensue if a seemingly weak system did not directly or indirectly impact on organizational performance.

This does not necessarily imply that performance audits are to be preferred. Practical problems are encountered when endeavouring to audit ends rather than means. Establishing representative, reliable and valid performance indicators for any public service is not easy and their interpretation is far from straight forward (Nutley and Smith, 1998). Performance and effectiveness are not straightforward concepts (Sicotte et al., 1998). In any organization they require us to specify performance for whom and effectiveness for whom. The need for stakeholder definitions of performance is particularly important in the public sector (Kanter and Summers, 1987). In the private sector we may be able to assume stakeholder satisfaction if there is long-term profitability. It is not possible to establish equivalent measures of bottom line performance in the public sector (Smith, 1996). In such circumstances it is not surprising that, as Walsh (1995, p. 94) comments: 'Since performance cannot be demonstrated, the nature of the management system became itself the mark of effectiveness'.

Performance audits within the HRM field tend to focus on HR outcomes rather than organizational performance. The HR outcomes may be judged by quantitative indicators (turnover and absenteeism rates) or by more qualitative indicators (such as staff satisfaction surveys). There may well be merit in auditing these intermediate performance indicators, especially if there is good evidence to support the assumption (see Figure 8.3) that good HR outcomes lead to good organizational performance. Storey (1989) is cautious about the possibility of demonstrating a causal linkage between different human resource practices and business performance because of the range of intervening variables. This has not prevented research (Patterson et al., 1997) sponsored by the Institute of Personnel Development (IPD) from concluding that:

> people management is not only critical to business performance: it also far outstrips emphasis on quality, technology, competitive strategy or research and development in its influence on the bottom line (West and Patterson, 1998, p. 22).

There are two aspects of the IPD research project which are salient for the purposes of this chapter. Firstly, the evidence for their conclusions comes from the private and not the public sector and we need to be cautious about assuming that the same relationship would hold true in the public sector. Secondly, even if such a connection were demonstrated in the public sector, the subsequent role of audit is still likely to centre on reviewing HRM systems rather than organizational outcomes. The IPD research report concludes with several recommendations concerning the need for good HRM systems – these include:

- senior managers should regularly review objectives, strategies and processes associated with people management practices;
- HRM practices should be reviewed across the organization in the following areas: recruitment and selection, appraisal, training, reward systems, design of jobs, and communication.

Thus in answering the question 'which HRM audit methodology?', the conclusion is that, in meeting the needs of a variety of stakeholders, it is unlikely that one type of audit is always to be preferred over the others. The audit role should be to check that good practices are being employed (however these are defined), and then to assess the impact of these processes on performance. Performance auditing does not replace the need for systems audits. The examination of performance without an analysis of processes would mean that audits could offer little in the way of organizational learning. Furthermore, despite the possible reinforcement of bureaucratization, it is doubtful whether the demands of public accountability would enable audits to move totally away from a systems approach.

The Effectiveness of HRM and the Efficacy of HRM Audits

There have been two important surveys of HRM effectiveness in the NHS during the 1990s. The first was conducted by Guest and Peccei (1992) and the second by the NHS Training Division (Tingey, 1994). Both of these studies entailed a form of audit of HRM effectiveness based upon a qualitative assessment of performance (that is the views of personnel managers and line managers).

The aim of the Guest and Peccei study was to develop and validate a qualitative measure of HRM effectiveness for use within the NHS. The study also explored any association between quantitative and qualitative measures of HRM effectiveness and the influence on effectiveness of a range of personnel inputs and processes. They found that NHS effectiveness was more highly rated on personnel administration than on policies typically associated with HRM. For example, HRM effectiveness was rated highest in the areas of industrial/employment relations and recruitment and selection. Performance was rated least effective on pay and rewards and design of jobs. The least effective areas are those associated with a human resource management ideology.

No clear relationship was found between the qualitative and quantitative outcome measures. The two sets of measures showed, at best, only a weak pattern of association. Effectiveness was not significantly related either to major structural factors such as size and type of unit, or to key characteristics of personnel such as the size, resourcing and professionalization of the personnel department. Effectiveness was found, instead, to be related to three main process variables. In order of their importance, the key predictors of good effectiveness ratings in the NHS were: i) the extent to which personnel policies are written down and formally agreed by members of the management team; ii) the extent to which personnel staff are seen as competent and responsive in the way they go about their business; and iii) the degree of influence which the personnel department has over major policy. These three core process variables were all found to have a strong and consistent positive impact on NHS effectiveness, as judged by qualitative outcome measures.

The NHS Training Division survey involved 18 NHS Trusts. The questionnaire followed the key competency areas adopted by the Personnel Standards Lead Body (PSLB) and the 33 survey questions were grouped into six broad areas: strategy and organization, resourcing, enhancement of individual and group performance, compensations and benefits, relations with employees, and work process in service delivery. A similar pattern of perceived effectiveness on personnel administration rather than the broader remit of an HRM ideology emerged. It was also clear that whilst personnel administration was considered effective, this was not seen as a priority by line managers. There were five personnel competence areas where importance for future success was rated high but where current capability of the personnel function to deliver was rated low. These five areas reflect the need for the NHS to shift towards more of an HRM ideology:

- enable the creation of an organization structure and work processes that maximize the performance of people at work;
- develop and maintain workforce planning to support current and future requirements;
- develop and maintain commitment of employees in times of change;
- promote effective communication within the organization;
- develop and maintain a reward strategy.

Conversely there were three personnel competence areas where importance for future success was rated as low but where current capability was judged to be high. These areas reflect a personnel administration orientation:

- recruit and select people in the organization;
- release people from the organization;
- pay contracted employees and others.

The message to emerge from both of the above studies is that qualitative assessments suggest that there needs to be a shift in emphasis away from personnel administration in the NHS towards the broader concerns of an HRM ideology. There are signs that the NHS is responding to this challenge. For example, as mentioned at the beginning of this chapter, the NHSiS launched a HR strategy in 1998. This strategy has the aim of ensuring that:

- changes in service delivery and care requiring new skills are underpinned by investment in education, training and development which balances the right of access and the responsibility of staff to maintain appropriate knowledge and skills levels;
- as change impacts on employment and jobs, an employee relation framework is created which gives staff the opportunity of real consultation, involvement and the ability to influence decision-making;
- a employment framework is put in place which offers employers flexibility and offers staff modern employment practices based on equality of opportunity;
- workforce planning supports the development of a workforce which is flexible and responsive and supports changes in service delivery;
- the environment in which staff work, is safe and secure, free from harassment and gives people the opportunity to manage their own health and fitness;
- pay and reward is affordable, fair and flexible. Any future system should be simple and should not require disproportionate effort to develop and maintain;
- the whole approach to the people in the NHS in Scotland is underpinned by a set of core values which are applied consistently across the Service.

A Scottish partnership forum is to be established to develop a framework for managing human resources in the NHSiS. There is also to be a Best Practice Steering Group to undertake research and provide advice on best practice in the delivery of support services.

Thus far this section has considered what we know about the effectiveness of HRM in the NHS. We now turn to the question of whether there is evidence that auditing HRM increases this effectiveness with the desired effect of improving the quality of health care serviced. The short answer to this question is that we lack such evidence.

Whilst there is evidence that HRM audit can signal ways of improving HRM effectiveness (Alberga et al. 1997; Nutley, 1998), there is little research evidence which explores the effect of HRM audit on subsequent organizational performance. Until such evidence becomes available the benefit of HRM audit in improving the quality of health care services remains an act of faith. Whatever the audit approach adopted there remains the danger that HRM audits do little to improve organizational performance. The fact that they are conducted at all could be due to the ritual of public sector management. Institutional theory (Meyer and Rowan, 1977) would suggest that the definition of the subject matter of audits according to the 'flavour' of the year indicates a ritualistic act.

In order to improve both the effectiveness of HRM and the contribution of HRM audits, we need to understand better how and what HRM interventions can help deliver more effective patient care. Insofar as we have any insight into this, it comes from the acute sector; we have only limited understanding of what HRM in primary care means. Moreover, HRM is only one of the organizational factors effecting subsequent performance (refer back to Figure 9.1). The beneficial effects of good HRM practices may be mitigated by other factors. For example, Flanagan (1998) argues that gaining the commitment of the workforce is the key to both effective HRM and effective organizational performance. He goes on to point out that gaining this commitment is not easy in the NHS when: a) direction, vision and goals are uncertain; b) management culture is driven by cost containment and constant adjustment of priorities.

Concluding Remarks

Much of the preceding chapter discusses how the way in which staff are deployed and managed is likely to effect the quality of health care. HRM is about ensuring that the right staff are employed in the right areas in the first place, and that their subsequent management results in committed and able employees. This should provide a solid foundation for quality of care. HRM audits try to ensure that this happens in practice. Thus they offer a specific tool for shaping one particular piece of the jigsaw that makes up health care quality.

We lack empirical evidence to confirm the causal linkage assumed by the above description. We do know that any form of audit is in danger of developing into a ritual which does little to improve organizational performance (Power, 1997). It may be that self-assessment (of the type encouraged by EFQM) rather that external scrutiny, might avoid the more ritualistic aspects of audit activity. These are important questions to which answers are still required.

Given that HRM audit is only one part of the quality jigsaw, it is important for there to be a dialogue between HRM audits and other quality initiatives in order to ensure the potential for synergy is realized.

References

Accounts Commission (1995), *Rewarding Work*, The Accounts Commission, Edinburgh.

Accounts Commission (1997), *Managing People: The Audit of Management Arrangements in Local Authorities*, Accounts Commission for Scotland, Edinburgh.

Alberga, T., Tyson, S. and Parsons, D. (1997), 'An Evaluation of the Investors in People Standard', *Human Resource Management Journal*, 7 (2), pp. 47–60.

Beer, M., Spector, B., Lawrence, P.R., Quinn, M.D. and Walton, R.E. (1984), *Managing Human Assets*, Free Press, New York.

Bowerman, M. (1996), 'Public Audit – Have We Got the Framework Right?' in Public Finance Foundation (ed.), *Adding Value? Audit and Accountability in the Public Services*, Chartered Institute of Public Finance and Accountancy, London.

British Quality Foundation (undated), *Towards Business Excellence*, British Quality Foundation, London.

Clark, J. (1994), 'Procedures and Consistency versus Flexibility and Commitment in Employee Relations: a comment on Storey', *Human Resource Management Journal*, 4 (1), pp. 79–81.

Collins, D.R. (1997), 'Human Resource Assessment – The Link to Mission', *Public Personnel Management*, 26 (1), pp. 1–6.

Davies, H.T.O. (1998), 'Performance Management using Health Outcomes: In search of instrumentality', editorial, *Journal of Evaluation in Clinical Practice*.

Davies, H.T.O. and Crombie, I.K. (1995), 'Assessing the Quality of Care: Measuring well supported processes may be more enlightening than monitoring outcomes', *British Medical Journal*, 311, p. 766.

Davies, H.T.O. and Crombie, I.K. (1997), 'Interpreting Health Outcome', *Journal of Evaluation in Clinical Practice*, 3 (3), pp. 187–200.

Dolenko, M. (1990), *Auditing Human Resources Management*, The Institute of Internal Auditors Research Foundation, Altamonte Springs, Florida.

Donabedian, A. (1980), *The Definition of Quality and Approaches to Its Assessment*, Health Administration Press, Ann Arbor, Michigan.

Flanagan, H. (1998), 'Literature Review of Organisational HRM Effectiveness', report for NHS project on Evaluating/Benchmarking HRM Effectiveness.

Guest, D. (1987), 'Human Resource Management and Industrial Relations', *Journal of Management Studies*, 24 (5), pp. 503–21.

Guest, D. and Peccei, R. (1992), *The Effectiveness of Personnel Management in the NHS*, NHS Personnel Development Division, London.

Kanter, R.M. and Summers, D.V. (1987), 'Doing Well While Doing Good: Dilemmas of performance measurement in nonprofit organisations and the need for a multiple constituency approach' in W.W. Powell (ed.), *The Non-Profit Sector: A Research Handbook*, Yale University Press, New Haven, Connecticut.

Legge, K. (1989), 'Human Resource Management: A critical analysis' in J. Storey (ed.), *New Perspectives on Human Resource Management*, Routledge, London.

Legge, K. (1995), 'HRM: Rhetoric, reality and hidden agendas' in J. Storey (ed.), *Human Resource Management*, Routledge, London.

Maxwell, R.J. (1992), 'Dimensions of Quality Revisited: From thought to action', *Quality in Health Care*, 1, pp. 171–7.

McGovern, P., Gratton, L., Stiles, P., Hope-Hailey, V. and Truss, C. (1997), 'Human Resource Management on the Line', *Human Resource Management Journal*, 7 (4), pp. 12–29.

Meyer, J.W. and Rowan, B. (1977), 'Institutional Organisations: Formal structure as myth and ceremony', *American Journal of Sociology*, 83, pp. 340–63.

Nutley, S. (1998), 'Naming the Beast: A taxonomy of public sector human resource management audits and an assessment of their strengths and weaknesses', working paper, University of St Andrews.

Nutley, S. and Smith, P. (1998), 'League Tables for Performance Improvement in Health Care', *Journal for Health Services Research and Policy*, 3 (1), pp. 50–8.

Open Business School (1992), *B884 Human Resource Strategies: Block 5 Assessing Human Resource Strategies*, The Open University, Milton Keynes.

Patterson, G.M., West, M.A., Lawthorn, R. and Nickell, S. (1997), *Impact of People Management Practices on Business Performance*, Institute of Personnel Development (IPD), London.

Power, M. (1994), *The Audit Explosion*, Demos, London.

Power, M. (1997), *The Audit Society: Rituals of Verification*, Oxford University Press, Oxford.

Sicotte, C., Champagne, F. and Contandriopoulour, A.P. (1998), 'A Conceptual Framework for the Analysis of Health Care Organizations' Performance', *Health Services Management Research*, 11, pp. 24–48.

Smith, P.E. (1996), *Measuring Outcome in the Public Sector*, Taylor & Francis, London.

Storey, J. (ed.) (1989), *New Perspectives on Human Resource Management*, Routledge, London.

Storey, J. (ed.) (1995), *Human Resource Management*, Routledge, London.

The Scottish Office (1998), *Towards a New Way of Working – the Plan for Managing People in the NHS in Scotland*, The Scottish Office, Department of Health, Edinburgh.

Tingey, S. (1994), *NHS Survey of Personnel Services Main Report*, NHS Training Division, Bristol.

Torrington, D. (1993), 'How Dangerous is HRM?: A reply to Hart', *Employee Relations*, 15 (5), pp. 40–53.

Treadway Commission (1992), *Internal Control – Integrated Framework*, Committee of Sponsoring Organizations of the Treadway Commission, London.

Ulrich, D. (1998), 'A New Mandate for Human Resources', *Harvard Business Review*, 76 (1), pp. 125–34.

Walsh, K. (1995), 'Quality through Markets: The new public services management' in A. Wilkinson and H. Willmott (eds), *Making Quality Critical*, Routledge, London.

West, M. and Patterson, M. (1998), 'Profitable Personnel', *People Management*, 8 January, pp. 28–31.

SECTION 3
USING PERFORMANCE INDICATORS

9 What Are We Counting with Hospital Episode Statistics (HES)?

RICHARD WILSON

Department of Public Health and Epidemiology, Medical School, University of Birmingham

Introduction

Hospital episode statistics (HES) were introduced in April 1987 to replace the 'ageing' hospital activity analysis and hospital inpatient enquiry. It was recognized that if management systems were to function effectively in the NHS, there had to be consistent and high quality data upon which decisions could be soundly based. The lack of such data was recognized by the Department of Health and Social Security (DHSS) in 1978, remarking at the time that the current collection of activity and financial statistics were 'unsatisfactory for planning work' (Steering Group on Health Services Information, 1982, p. 7). The Resource Allocation Working Party (RAWP) had earlier stated, in 1976, that there was a 'pressing need for improvement in the data routinely collected'. The major change was to move away from the recording of 'deaths and discharges' to the consultant episode, that is 'the time a patient spends in the care of one consultant' (ibid., p. 26). This measure was decided upon as it could be used to determine both the health care experience of the patient, as well as the workloads of consultants and medical facilities.

When the HES system was introduced, it was criticized for not being relevant to public health, lacking in appropriate patient identifiers, socio-demographic details and clinical information (Knox, 1987). However, despite these criticisms in the last 10 years, HES has been used to inform much of national and regional policies as well as in epidemiological studies. HES was

Managing Quality: Strategic Issues in Health Care Management, H.T.O. Davies, M. Malek, A.R. Neilson, M. Tavakoli (eds), Ashgate Publishing Ltd, 1999.

used in the development of the new capitation based resource allocation formula (Carr-Hill, Hardman et al. , 1994). It became the unit of production for the internal market and as such the consultant episode was at the heart of the contracting process (Reeves, 1994), and is the key element of the costed Healthcare Resource Groups (HRGs). In 1998, the focus of health care in the UK is moving away from competitive purchasing towards health-focused commissioning challenging the future role of the FCE.

There is now a need to review the situation and consider the efficacy of the system as it now stands. This review needs to consider what is now being counted under the auspices of the FCE, how it is being used, and the quality of coding. This paper considers these issue from a perspective of a review of 10 years of HES data, from its introduction in 1987 to March 1997, for the West Midlands region, and from data in published studies. Analyses will be presented on the quality of coding measured in terms of completeness, accuracy and precision (McKee, 1993). Also, the issue of 'episode inflation', that is the occurrence of secondary episodes, will be explored. Discussion will focus on how these factors could influence policy decisions and the provision of health care.

Completeness

How complete a data set is can be defined in two ways: i) internal completeness; that is, how many episodes in the data set have, at the very least, the core data items of date of birth, gender and main diagnosis completed after a specified period; and ii) coverage; how many episodes have been 'lost' during data collection.

Accuracy

The accuracy of data items within a data set is determined by the means of recording the information, be it either directly into a computer in response to questions or via the inputting of paper returns, and the encoding of data into standardized classifications. Inaccuracy can enter a data set from the very outset of recording. A patient may respond incorrectly to a question or the person recording their answers may mark the wrong box. Such human errors are common and well recorded (Wyatt, 1994). Differences can also occur in the interpretation of a patient's symptoms. In a study of hospital databases, Cleary et al. (1994) observed that when reviewing the primary diagnoses of 18 cases, two consultants only agreed on 11 occasions. Furthermore, even if the diagnosis is valid and the patient has responded correctly to the questions asked of them, the data inputter may make an error when keying in the data.

Another example of the type of inaccuracies that can occur is given by the recording of postcode of residency. For a postcode to be matched to an electoral ward or health authority, the patient must first have knowledge of their postcode and have remembered it correctly. Ben-Schlomo and Chaturvedi (1995) reported errors of 2.4 per cent in matching completed postcodes to an electoral ward. Carr-Hill and Hardman (1994) reported another type of error that can create anomalous results when using postcodes in any statistical modelling process, namely the use of dummy or bin postcodes. Many service contracts now require that the HES be completed before settlement is made, and hence clerks are under pressure to make sure every data field is 100 per cent complete. Therefore, any patient who does not know their postcode may be dumped into a dummy or bin postcode. The result of this is to exaggerate any measure produced for the geographical area in which that postcode falls, or the recording of 'levels of homeless' people.

Precision

The degree of precision used in recording information is determined by how fully an event is described within a data set. The data set could be said to be complete if the main diagnosis field is filled in. It would be accurate if the patient's condition was correctly identified. However, the degree of precision would be low if additional information regarding the cause of injury or co-morbidities present were not recorded.

The disease (International Classification of Diseases Ninth and Tenth revision – ICD9 and ICD10) and operative and procedure (Office of Population, Census and Surveys Version 4 – OPCS4) classifications were chosen to lend precision and standardization to the recording of patient characteristics: however, this is not always the case. The inclusion of catch-all categories, in particular the last digit '.9', 'unspecified' code in both ICD and OPCS4 can be abused, leading to imprecision in the data set. The same can be said when 'incorrect' alternative codes, such as 'retention of urine' are used as a principal diagnosis for a patient undergoing a prostatectomy (McKee, 1993). However, work by Williams et al. (1994) into the contrasting levels of diabetes recorded in the hospital activity analysis and HES, found that the introduction of ICD9 and the HES had possibly led to greater precision. They report that over three years from 1988/89 to 1990/91 admission rates for ICD 250.0 – diabetes with no mention of complications – fell from 61.6 per cent to

38.0 per cent of all diabetes-related episodes. They state that one of the possible reasons for this could be 'an increase in the precision of coding' and in particular the 'improved recording of complications in discharge summaries' (Williams et al. 1994, p. 169). The review of published data found rates of imprecision in the range of 5–59 per cent.

Episode Inflation

An issue unique to this data set, which is related to precision, is the concern over the interpretation of the consultant episode, the basic building block of the minimum data set. The consultant episode is defined as the 'time a patient spends continuously in the care of one consultant or general practitioner' (Steering Group on Health Services Information, 1985, p. 7). It was designed to give a uniform measure of activity across the Health Service, but since the introduction of the NHS reforms in 1991, there has been growing concern that hospitals are abusing the definition to their commercial advantage. The Radical Statistic Group first raised the concept of increasing numbers of episodes for the same number of admissions, or discharges, in 1992, in their examination of the first six months of the NHS reforms. They stated that the reforms were likely to 'provide a financial incentive for more complete reporting' of a patient's treatment (Radical Statistics Health Group, 1992, p. 706), a view which was supported by Clarke and Tinsley, who questioned their local provider's estimated level of activity for the next financial year. They reported that across medical specialties, a slight improvement in the 'accuracy of recording completed consultant episodes per discharge can result in a substantial increase in apparent activity', thus giving rise to the 'perverse incentives within the internal market' (Clarke and Tinsley, 1992, p. 987) for providers to optimize their income without increasing their workload.

Pollock and Majeed (1993) dispute the belief that providers are playing the system, stating that this view is derived solely from the experience of the United States. Indeed, there is little evidence from the Health Service that the providers are systematically massaging the figures. The only reported suggestion of any such 'fiddling' of the figures by a provider came from a Trust's outgoing finance director. However, her comments were not concerned with the issue of episode inflation, rather the interpretation of the Trust's performance statistics (Hunter, 1996).

Despite the concerns raised, little has been reported on the extent of the problem. Seng et al. investigated the issue in their local provider (1993). They examined the medical records of patients who had not had a co-terminous admission and consultant episode. They discovered that multiple episodes arose as the result of transfers to other departments, for investigations or treatment, and back again, typically resulting in three episodes. Multiple admissions were also occurring for planned treatments such as blood transfusions. They concluded that such practices suggest the possibility that the reported increases in the workload of their provider unit may not be 'all that they seem', and that consultant episodes 'should not be equated with the number of patients treated' (Seng, Lessof et al., 1993, p. 17).

Both Seng and Clarke support the replacement of the episode. They favour a new activity measure that would be better suited to the post-reform NHS, which would curtail the 'excesses' of the provider units, but neither suggest where one might find such a measure routinely collected within the Health Service.

Data

The primary data set is all finished consultant episodes undertaken in NHS Hospitals in the West Midlands region from April 1987 to March 1997. In these 10 years, this totals some 10,469,843 FCEs. The numbers of FCEs have risen by an average of 4.2 per cent year on year. The comparative source of hospital activity data chosen was the Financial Return 22, which records the number of inpatient episodes by each provider across 40 specialties (CIPFA, 1995).

In addition to the analysis of HES, a review of published studies using HES was undertaken. This review identified 14 journal and conference papers from a wide range of fields which had either used HES to report on variations in treatment patterns or examined the quality of HES.

Data Analysis

Completeness

Internal completeness The completion of individual fields remains patchy. The proportion of incomplete fields reported ranges between 0.0 per cent and 33 per cent (see Table 9.1). The degree of completion tends to be highest in the clinical fields of main diagnosis and operation.

To gain a better understanding of the levels of completion across the major

Table 9.1   Published completion rates for HES

Author	Year	Area	Condition	Variable	Completeness	Accuracy	Precision
Parkin et al. (1993)	1987–8	Health Authority	Day cases	Main diagnosis and/or main operation	99.99%		
Smith et al. (1991)	1987–8	3 hospitals	Joint replacements	Main procedure			76%
McKee & Petticrew (1993)	1988–9	Sample of England data set	All conditions in 13 specialties	Main diagnosis	91–100%		
Sudell et al. (1991)	1988–9	Hospital and 10% regional sample data set	General medicine	Discharge destination	75%		
Black (1995)	1987–91	Regional Health Authority	Glue ear	Main procedure	90–97%		
Carr–Hill et al. (1994)	1990–1	England	All conditions	Postcode			
Cleary et al. (1994)	1990–1	Hospital	General medicine, General surgery and obstetrics	Main diagnosis	67–89%		
Yeoh & Davies (1993)	1990–1	Hospital	Paediatrics	Main diagnosis	100%	95%	
				Postcode	97.6%		
				Sex	99.2%		
Ben–Schlomo and Chaturvedi (1995)	1991–2	Regional Health Authority	Coronary artery bypass graft	Main operation	88.5%		
Walshe, Harrison, and Renshaw (1993)	1991–2	Hospital	Urology	Main diagnosis	95%		
Dixon et al. (1996)	1991–3	Two hospitals (A&B)	All conditions	Main diagnosis		54%(A) 70%(B)	41%(A) 59%(B)
				Main operation		71%(A) 79%(B)	52%(A) 69%(B)
Pantin (1994)	1992–3	Health Authority	Gastroscopies	Main operation		59%	
Chenet and McKee (1996)	1993–4	Health Authority	Other general symptoms	Main diagnosis	98.6%		
Maheswaran (1997)	1994–5	England	All admissions[1]	Primary			95.2%
				Postcode	89.9%		
				Sex	99.7%	99.4%[2]	

Notes

1   All admissions episode order number = 1.
2   Indeterminate sex.

fields the proportion of West Midland FCEs with specified fields completed was calculated for the period April 1987 to March 1997. The completion of core data items of sex and age is high, averaging 99.9 per cent (see Table 9.2). The same is not true of the main diagnosis codes. In the first year of the data set, 1987-8 there was a completion rate of 75.9 per cent (699,013/920,955). However, this has been improving, and the completion rate has risen to 91.9 per cent (1,255,528/1,267,502) in 1996–7. The other data items of interest have differing levels of completeness. Admission method, discharge destination, patient classification, postcode and specialty all had high completion rates of between 99.2 and 100 per cent.

Table 9.2   The internal completeness of HES measured in terms of the proportion of those fields completed

Field	1987/8	1988/9	1989/90	1990/1	1991/2	1992/3	1993/4	1994/5	1995/6	1996/7
Age	100.0	100.0	100.0	100.0	100.0	100.0	100.0	100.0	100.0	100.0
Sex	100.0	100.0	100.0	100.0	100.0	99.9	100.0	100.0	99.2	99.2
Admission method	100.0	100.0	100.0	100.0	100.0	99.9	99.9	99.2	100.0	100.0
Discharge destination	100.0	100.0	100.0	100.0	100.0	100.0	100.0	100.0	99.2	99.2
Hospital	100.0	100.0	100.0	100.0	100.0	100.0	100.0	100.0	100.0	100.0
Main diagnosis	75.9	89.5	90.5	90.0	93.9	96.3	96.6	88.9	90.3	90.1
Main procedure	17.8	42.0	42.1	41.3	44.7	46.9	47.2	49.1	50.0	51.1
Patient classification	100.0	100.0	100.0	100.0	100.0	100.0	100.0	100.0	99.2	99.2
Postcode	100.0	100.0	99.3	100.0	99.9	100.0	100.0	100.0	100.0	100.0
Specialty	100.0	100.0	100.0	100.0	100.0	100.0	100.0	100.0	99.2	99.2

Source: West Midlands HES Data, April 1987–March 1997.

Coverage

The completeness of coverage is far more difficult to measure. Hospitals are duty bound to record each episode of consultant care, hence it should be complete, but it is not. Majeed and Pollock (1995) discovered anomalies in the treatment of ischaemic heart disease using angiographs and reperfusion treatment. They discovered that despite the fact that an angiograph is always carried out before reperfusion treatment, that there were more episodes of the latter. This anomaly was due to the under-coding of angiography by the local provider unit. Similar shortfalls were observed by Lyons and Gumpet (1990). Carr-Hill et al. (1994) report that, when comparing HES data to corporate return data, which is compiled independently of HES, there is often either a slight excess or shortfall in regional episode counts. However, in one instance they observed an excess of 28 per cent in HES.

To investigate coverage three West Midlands hospitals were chosen to reflect the range of providers and their FCE counts across five specialties were compared to the corporate contracting data as recorded on the Financial Return 22. This was carried out to measure any 'leakage' in the data set, in a similar fashion to that of Carr-Hill and Hardman (1994). The comparison gives a confusing picture (see Table 9.3). It is generally believed that the HES data undercounts true activity; however, when compared to the providers' declared workload, HES is higher in most specialties, apart from surgery.

Table 9.3   The coverage of HES as the measured percentage divergence of HES from FR22 data for three providers across a range of specialties

	Paediatrics	Geriatrics	Other medical	Surgical specialties	Maternity	All specialties
Birmingham Heartlands	8.9	-19.7	61.1	-12.5	-34.1	38.9
North Staffs Hospital Centres	38.3	100.0[1]	4.0	-25.0	-0.0	99.1
Worcester Royal Infirmary	-14.2	0.3	0.04	-31.2	-35.0	-1.94

Note

1   HES records 53 episodes but FR22 records 0 episodes.

Sources: West Midlands HES April 1995–March 1996; CIPFA Database 1995.

Accuracy

It is difficult to report on the accuracy of any data item beyond its face value, without resorting to case notes. The published data on the inaccuracy of items which report a range from 0.6 per cent to 59 per cent across various fields all come from small localized studies. Such studies would be unfeasible to carry out on the 10 million FCEs of the West Midlands HES. However, there is a proxy in the Healthcare Resource Groups which contains four measures reporting on the validity of the data recorded.

* U02 – primary procedure invalid for grouping: the procedure is either invalid or not usable for primary position;
* U03 – primary diagnosis invalid for grouping: the diagnosis is either invalid or not usable for primary position;

- U04 – age outside range: it is either blank or invalid, that is, over 130;
- U05 – age conflict: age on record is not valid for diagnosis or procedure.

The proportion of records assigned to these codes is reported for the six years of West Midlands data which had been grouped into HRGs, April 1991/2– March 1996/7. The levels of accuracy measured by the HRG U-codes is generally high (see Table 9.4). The worst fields are invalid diagnoses fields (U2). These levels are due, in the main, to one provider whose error rate for this code is consistently over 15 per cent. This is different to U3 – missing procedure codes – where the error rate remains fairly consistent across all units, around 0.5 per cent. The accuracy for age-related fields is high (U4– U5), with few errors being reported.

Table 9.4   The accuracy of West Midlands HES, as recorded by the percentage of episodes coded with a HRG Version 2 code U02–U05

Year	U02	U03	U04	U05
1991/2	0.40	2.01	0.09	0.00
1992/3	0.81	0.75	0.06	0.00
1993/4	1.13	0.85	0.01	0.00
1994/5	1.33	0.73	0.01	0.00
1995/6	1.13	0.70	0.01	0.00
1996/7	1.18	0.48	0.01	0.00

Source: West Midlands HES April 1991–March 1997.

Precision

Precision is reported much less in the literature than completion and accuracy, and when it is, it tends to be lower. Again, like accuracy, precision is also difficult to measure without recourse to patient notes. This study uses selected ICD10 codes taken from chapter XVIII (R00–R99) symptoms, sign and abnormal clinical and laboratory findings, not elsewhere classified as a proxy for the degree of precision. If the precision of coding was improving it would be expected that these codes would be on the decline. For the purpose of investigating trends over time, the ICD10 codes were matched to ICD9 codes for the years April 1987–March 1995. The tenth revision of the ICD classification superseded the ninth revision in April 1995. Renal Colic (N23) was included in the groupings as it had previously been part of the symptoms involving urinary system in ICD9.

The use of 'general' conditions was, up to the introduction of ICD10 in 1995/6, steadily rising, to a high of 7.64 per cent FCEs, in 1994/5 (see Table 9.5). However, the trend changed with the introduction of ICD10. For three of the categories (symptoms involving circulatory and respiratory systems, R00–R09, and symptoms involving digestive system and abdomen, R10–19, symptoms involving skin and subcutaneous tissue) the trend has continued steadily upwards. For the other conditions there have been huge swings either upward or downward. In the urinary category, the downward shift is due apparently to the 'curing' of both renal colic (N23) and retention of urine (R33). These conditions dropped from 1,982 and 3,206 FCES, respectively, to 0 in 1995/6. The ill-defined causes of morbidity and mortality have dropped away, reflecting a possible improvement in the precision of coding, as no longer are 1.2 per cent FCEs being recorded as 'other unknown and unspecified cause' as had been the case under ICD9.

An additional measure of precision is the coding of co-mordidities and additional procedures. This can be measured by examining the depth of coding of both diagnosis and procedures. There is room for up to seven diagnoses and five operations to be coded in HES. The depth of coding of main diagnosis has improved over the years (see Figure 9.1). In 1987/8, only 11.8 per cent of

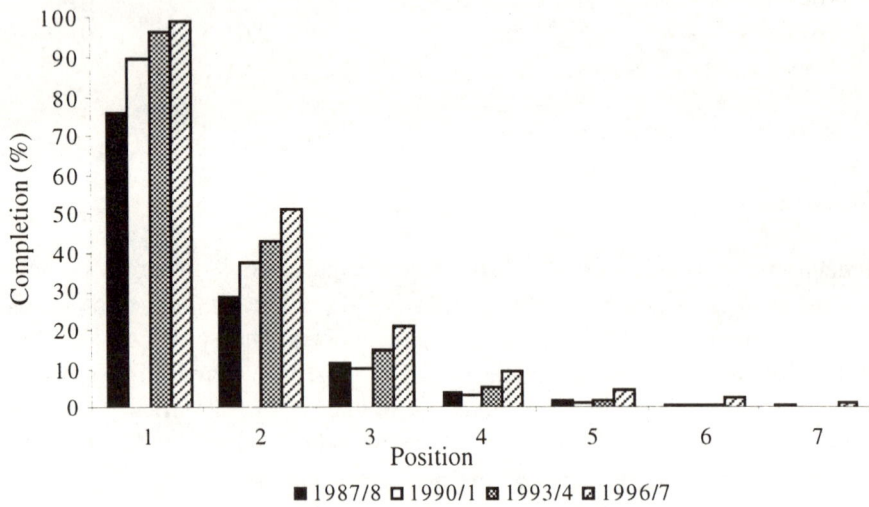

Figure 9.1   Depth of coding for main and additional diagnosis codes, for the years 1987/8, 1990/1, 1993/4 and 1996/7

Table 9.5   The percentage of episodes coded with a 'general' condition in the main diagnosis field

Conditions	ICD10 codes	1987/8	1988/9	1989/90	1990/1	1991/2	1992/3	1993/4	1994/5	1995/6	1996/7
Symptoms involving circulatory and respiratory systems	R00–R09	0.96	1.22	1.21	1.22	1.25	1.40	1.54	1.53	1.60	1.74
Symptoms involving digestive system and abdomen	R10–R19	1.85	2.16	2.23	2.11	2.16	2.32	2.35	2.31	2.09	2.13
Symptoms involving skin and subcutaneous tissue	R20–R23 and R60	0.07	0.08	0.09	0.09	0.09	0.11	0.11	0.13	0.13	0.13
Symptoms involving nervous and musclosketal systems	R25–R29	0.02	0.03	0.03	0.04	0.04	0.04	0.04	0.04	0.11	0.11
Symptoms involving urinary system inc. renal colic	R30–R39 and N23	0.47	0.56	0.60	0.56	0.60	0.61	0.58	0.68	0.07	0.07
Symptoms involving cognition, perception and emotional state	R40–R46	0.05	0.07	0.07	0.06	0.07	0.08	0.08	0.08	0.12	0.12
Symptoms involving speech and voice	R47–R49 and R51	0.05	0.05	0.05	0.04	0.04	0.04	0.04	0.04	0.03	0.03
General symptoms	R50–R64	0.85	1.04	1.08	1.04	1.09	1.14	1.18	1.25	0.71	0.69
Ill–defined causes of mortality and morbidity	R68, R69 R99	0.63	0.42	0.35	0.18	0.22	0.95	1.72	1.23	0.02	0.03
Overall		4.96	5.63	5.71	5.34	5.57	6.67	7.64	7.29	4.88	5.04

Source: West Midlands HES April 1991–March 1997.

episodes had supplementary or co-morbidities coded to the third position out of seven, by 1996/7 the number had almost doubled to 21.3 per cent. Similarly, the depth of coding of main and additional procedures has improved (see Figure 9.2). In 1987/8, only 9.2 per cent of episodes had an additional procedure coded, by 1996/7, 23.8 per cent episodes listed at least two procedures.

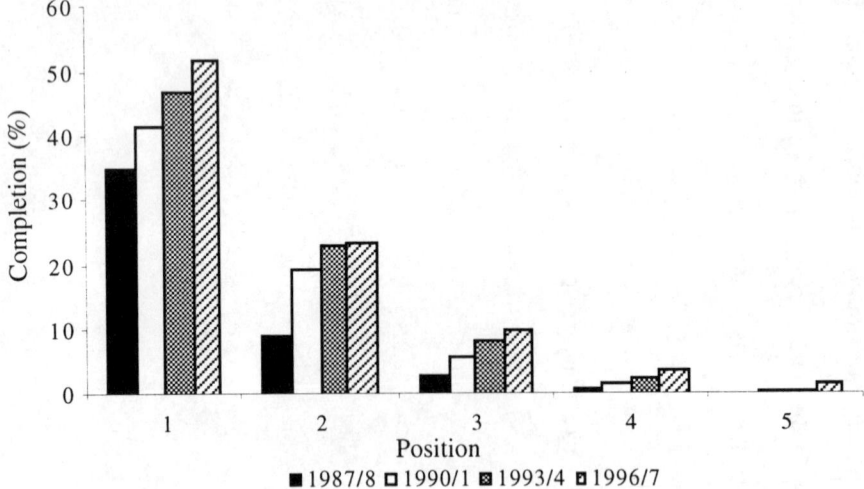

Figure 9.2   Depth of coding for main and additional procedure codes, for the years 1987/8, 1990/1, 1993/4 and 1996/7

Episode Inflation

To measure the recording of secondary episodes, the West Midlands HES data was filtered first by patient classification, to exclude those episodes which were either day cases or regular attenders, to leave ordinary inpatient episodes. The data set was then filtered into either admission episodes or secondary episodes by the episode order number. Where the episode order number was 1 it was declared an admission and greater than 1 a secondary episode. A ratio was then calculated for admissions to secondary episodes.

The ratio of admissions to secondary episodes for emergency admissions has increased since 1987/8, from there being 107 episodes for every 100 admissions to, in 1996/7, 115 episodes for every 100 admissions (see Figure 9.3). The ratio has increased more rapidly in the last three years. For elective admissions the ratio has remained steady, with only a slight rise in the last year.

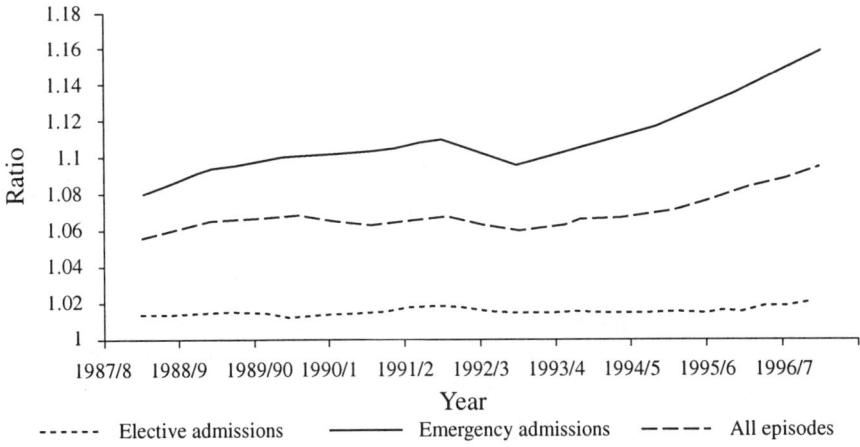

Figure 9.3 **Episode inflation, the ratio of admission episodes to secondary episodes for elective, emergency and all episodes, for the years 1987/8 to 1996/7, for the West Midlands**

Conclusion

This study found similar results regarding the quality of HES as previous studies. The completeness of the individual fields was generally high at around 99 per cent. The highest levels of non-completion are recorded in the main operation code fields. This is caused by the lack of a default 'no operation' code in the HES. If an operation code is blank, it has duplicity of meanings. It can mean either that there was no operation performed or that there was no record of an operation, if one was carried out.

The coverage of HES is more difficult to validate. This work gave the example of comparing HES to FR22 data. Both data sets are generated by the same organization and claim to count the same workload, but are dramatically different. There is no consistency in the under- or over-counting, other than that HES seems to, at least for these providers, under-count surgery. Some of this variation could be explained by the definition of consultant and specialty of treatment. This could be especially true in the medical specialties, where one is likely to find general medicine consultants with an interest in a sub-specialty working in a ward dedicated to that sub-specialty. In HES, any FCEs attributed to that consultant would be recorded under general medicine, where as the FR22 data may record that as activity in the ward's sub-specialty. However, that would not explain the large shortfall in HES for the surgical specialties. It is possible that this work reflects less failings of HES than failings in the recording of FR22 data, especially considering the 38.9 per cent under-count observed for Birmingham Heartlands. More work needs to undertaken to assess which data set is the more reliable and whether it is worth collecting the FR22.

It is difficult to report on the accuracy and precision within the HES data set without using patient records. The accuracy of HES appears fairly robust, that is, the data recorded fulfils the requirements for that field. The HRG codes report error rates around 1.2 per cent. However, that is not to say that the information reported is correct. It would be an impossible task to audit each record referring back to the patient's case notes. Indeed, sometimes when this has been attempted in even small-scale studies it has not been achieved (Cleary, 1994; Seng et al., 1993). The published accuracy rates range from 5 per cent to 46 per cent for main diagnosis and 21 per cent to 29 per cent for main operation. It is important to consider these rates when studying specific diseases or conditions using this data set.

It is difficult to say conclusively if HES has become any more precise over the years. Depth of coding has improved dramatically, but has it become any more detailed? From the work carried out here on the use of 'general' codes, it cannot conclusively be said to be improving. The drop in the overall proportion of 'general' codes may be an artefact of the introduction of ICD10 and the problems matching it to ICD9. In addition to the problems seen with ICD10, the procedure codes are becoming dated, as the last revision was over five years ago. A review of the procedure codes is currently being undertaken but it is unlikely that any revisions suggested would be in place before April 2000.

Over the years, it is also becoming apparent that episode inflation is rising steadily, driven by the increasing use of secondary episodes in emergency admissions. It is surprising that the ratio has not increased for elective admissions as, with short stay procedures transferring to day cases, the more complex cases remain. This might imply that there has been little change in the unbundling of elective episodes. This is different to results reported by Soderlund et al. (1997) who report a decreasing ratio across the years 1991–94. However, they do not exclude day cases from their calculations. The inclusion of these patient groups will deflate the ratio as they are single episode admissions.

The effect of data quality on the application of HES in decision-making is difficult to predict. If one assumes the errors are random, then the rates observed should not pose a great problem in planning. If the errors are systematic to a specific specialty or unit then this could lead to the misallocation of resources. The purpose to which the data are going to be applied must be taken into context when considered the effect of data quality. For general variations in the uptake of hospital services, the precision of main diagnosis codes will not be important. However, this would not be true for a descriptive study into a specific condition. The advice would be to proceed with caution and to consider the rates produced locally to any comparators published elsewhere. Indeed HES has been successfully used in a number of epidemiological and public health studies (Black, 1995; Hyndman et al., 1994; Majeed and Cook, 1996; Mulholland et al., 1996; Walters et al., 1994 and 1996; Weinberg, 1995).

Of perhaps greater importance to the health care planner is the issue of episode inflation. It is not clear yet what is happening to drive up the ratio, but it alone is responsible for an annual rise in 'productivity' of 0.5 per cent. More investigations need to be carried out to see how this rise in 'productivity' is generated and funded, especially, as the ratio varies considerably amongst providers. It is possible, that providers with elevated ratios, are placing an inflated demand on resources through the generation of excessive extra contractual referrals, to the detriment of other providers in the same health authority.

HES is currently at a transition point: with the end of the internal market there is likely to be less focus on the data set for performance monitoring, at least to the degree undertaken for contract monitoring. However, the exposure HES received as the currency of the internal market now means that more people are aware of the information it can provide. This is especially true in the field of public health, both academic and in the NHS. Unfortunately, this interest comes at the time of the greatest commercialization of access to the data, which could impose the greatest restrictions on its use. It is hoped that the central role HES plays in the new performance indicators proposed by the government's white paper *The New NHS, Modern and Dependable* (NHSE, 1998), will mean that improvements in coding will continue and more consistent definitions for FCE developed. Bearing in mind the caveats raised by this work, the HES data set provides a very valuable resource, which deserves talking up in terms of its quality and vast applications. Only by making the data set work for the health service, will the health service regard the efforts required to collect HES worthwhile.[1]

Note

1   The author would like to acknowledge the continued support of the West Midlands Public Health Levy and the West Midlands Regional Information Department for access to the HES data.

References

Ben-Schlomo, Y. and Chaturvedi, N. (1995), 'Assessing Equity in Access to Health Care Provision in the UK: Does where you live affect your chances of getting a coronary artery bypass graft?', *Journal of Epidemiology and Community Health*, 49, pp. 200–4.

Black, N. (1995), 'Surgery for glue ear: the English epidemic wanes', *Journal of Epidemiology and Community Health*, 49, pp. 234–7.

Carr-Hill, R.A., Hardman, G., Martin, S., Peacock, S., Sheldon, T.A. and Smith, P. (1994), *A Formula for Distributing NHS Revenues Based on Small Area Use of Hospital Beds*, Centre for Health Economics, University of York, York.

Chenet, L. and McKee, M. (1996), 'Challenges of Monitoring Use of Secondary Care at Local Level: A study based in London, UK', *Journal of Epidemiology and Community Heath*, 50, pp. 359–65.

CIPFA (1995), *Provider Database: Activity Cost Analysis*, Chameleon Press, London.

Clarke, A. and Tinsley, P. (1992), 'Completed consultant episodes increase but hospital discharges decrease', *British Medical Journal*, 304, p. 987.

Cleary, R., Beard, R., Coles, J., Devlin, B., Hopkins, A., Schumacher, D. and Wickings, I. (1994), 'Comparative Hospital Databases: Value for management and quality', *Quality in Health Care*, 3, pp. 3–10.

Dixon, J., Sanderson, C., Elliott, P., Walls, P., Petticrew, M. and Jones, J. (1996), 'Estimating the Accuracy of Clinical Codes Recorded on Hospital Episode Statistics Data', *The Society for Social Medicine: 40th Annual Scientific Meeting*, University of Dundee.

Hunter, H. (1996), 'Finance Director Quits NHS with Claims of "Fiddle" Ethos', *Health Service Journal*, 2 May, p. 8.

Hyndman, S.J., Williams, D.R.R. et al. (1994), 'Rates of Admission to Hospital for Asthma', *British Medical Journal*, 308, pp. 1596–600.

Knox, E.G. (ed.) (1987), *Health-care Information. Report of a joint working group of the Körner Committee on Health Services Information and the Faculty of Community Medicine*, Occasional Papers, Nuffield Provincial Hospitals Trust, London.

Lyons, C. and Gumpet, R. (1990), 'Medical Audit Data: Counting is not enough', *British Medical Journal*, 300, pp. 1563–6.

Maheswaran, R. (1997), 'HES and Small Area Epidemiology', *HES, the conference*, IBM South Bank, London.

Majeed, F.A. and Cook, D.G. (1996), 'Age and Sex Differences in the Management of Ischaemic Heart Disease', *Public Health*, 110, pp. 7–12.

Majeed, F.A. and Pollock, A. (1995), 'Set Piece', *Health Service Journal*, 105 (5444), pp. 28–9.

McKee, M. (1993), 'Routine data: a resource for clinical audit', *Quality in Health Care*, 2, pp. 104–11.

McKee, M. and Petticrew, M. (1993), 'Disease Staging – a case-mix system for purchasers?', *Journal for Public Health Medicine*, 15 (1), pp. 25–3.

Mulholland, C., Harding, N., Bradley, S. and Stevenson, M. (1996), 'Regional Variations in the Utilization Rate of Vaginal and Abdominal Hysterectomies in the United Kingdom', *Journal of Public Health Medicine*, 18 (4), pp. 400–5.

NHS Executive (1998), *The New NHS, Modern and Dependable: A National Framework for Assessing Performance*, Department of Health, London.

Pantin, C.F.A. (1994), 'Clinical Information in the NHS – the why, what and how', *Journal of the Royal College of Physicans of London*, 28 (2), pp. 163–7.

Parkin, D., Hutchieson, A., Philips, P. and Coates, J. (1993), 'A Comparison of Disease Related Groups and Ambulatory Visit Groups on Day Surgery', *Health Trends*, 25 (1), pp. 41–4.

Pollock, A. and Majeed, A. (1993), 'Consultant Episodes', *British Medical Journal*, 306, pp. 141–2.

Radical Statistics Health Group (1992), 'NHS Reforms: The first six months – proof of progress or a statistical smokescreen', *British Medical Journal*, 304, pp. 705–9.

Reeves, C. (1994), 'Perspectives on Purchasing: Cabbages and Things', *Health Service Journal*, 3 March, pp. 29–30.

Rowe, R.G. and Brewer, W. (1972), *Hospital Activity Analysis*, Butterworths, London.

Seng, C., Lessof, L. and McKee, M. (1993), 'Who's on the Fiddle?', *Health Service Journal*, 7 January, pp. 16–17.

Smith, S.H., Kershaw, C., Thomas, I.H. and Botha, J.L. (1991), 'PIS and DRGs: Coding inaccuracies and their consequences for resource management', *Journal of Public Health Medicine*, 13 (1), pp. 40–1.

Soderlund, N., Csaba, I., Gray, A., Milne, R. and Raftery, J. (1997), 'Impact of the NHS Reforms on English Hospital Productivity: An analysis of the first three years', *British Medical Journal*, 315, pp. 1126–9.

Steering Group on Health Services Information (1982), *First Report to the Secretary of State*, National Health Service, Department of Health and Social Security, London.

Steering Group on Health Services Information (1985), *Supplement to the First and Fourth Reports to the Secretary of State*, National Health Service, Department of Health and Social Security, London.

Sudell, A.J., Horner, J.S., Jolly, U. and Pain, C.H. (1991), 'Length of Stay in General Medicine Beds; Implications for the NHS White Paper of variance within one performance indicator', *Journal of Public Health Medicine*, 13 (2), pp. 88–9.

Walshe, K., Harrison, N. and Renshaw, M. (1993), 'Comparison of the Quality of Patient Data Collected by Hospital and Departmental Computer Systems', *Health Trends*, 25 (3), pp. 105–8.

Walters, S., Griffiths, R.K. and Ayres, J.G. (1994), 'Temporal Association Between Hospital Admissions for Asthma in Birmingham and Ambient Levels of Sulphur Dioxide and Smoke', *Thorax*, 49, pp. 133–40.

Watson, J.P., Cowen, P. and Lewis, R.A. (1996), 'The Relationship Between Asthma Admission Rates, Routes of Admission, and Socio-economic Deprivation', *European Respiratory Journal*, 9, pp. 2087–93.

Weinberg, J. (1995), 'The Impact of Ageing upon the Need for Medical Beds: A Monte-Carlo simulation', *Journal of Public Health Medicine*, 17 (3), pp. 290–6.

Williams, D.R.R., Anthony, P., Young, R.J. and Tomlinson, S. (1994), 'Interpreting Hospital Admissions Data Across the Körner Divide – the Example Of Diabetes In the North-Western Region', *Diabetic Medicine*, 11 (2), pp. 166–9.

Wyatt, J.C. (1994), 'Clinical Data Systems, Part 1: Data and medical records', *The Lancet*, 344, pp. 1543–7.

Yeoh, C. and Davies, H. (1993), 'Clinical Coding: Completeness and accuracy when doctors take it on', *British Medical Journal*, 306, p. 972.

10 Clinical Outcomes Indicators in Scotland: Lessons and Prospects

STEVE KENDRICK,[1] DAVID CLINE[2] AND ALAN FINLAYSON[1]

1   *ISD Scotland*
2   *CRAG Secretariat*

Introduction

It is now over five years since the first pilot clinical outcome indicators were produced by ISD Scotland for the Clinical Outcomes Working Group of the National Health Service in Scotland. Since then over 30 indicators have been published at hospital, Trust or Health Board level in five reports.

This chapter takes stock of this experience and its lessons for how best to use the monitoring of clinical outcomes to improve the quality of health care. The key message is that the indicators do not provide proof in themselves that one hospital provides better care than another but rather that they provide useful evidence for the Health Service to use alongside other sources of insight and information in working to do things better.

Background

A Brief History of the Indicators

Scotland has been able to publish clinical outcome indicators because of the coincidence of the development of the policy drive to produce and publish them and the availability of information systems on which they could be based. The will and the way were both present.

In terms of policy, a working group set up by the Scottish Office had

Managing Quality: Strategic Issues in Health Care Management, H.T.O. Davies, M. Tavakoli, M. Malek, A.R. Neilson (eds), Ashgate Publishing Ltd, 1999.

recommended in 1989 that clinical outcome indicators be developed by the Health Service in Scotland (Clinical Resource and Audit Group, 1989). In 1992, the Clinical Outcomes Working Group was set up by CRAG (see Box) to recommend how this should be done (Clinical Outcomes Working Group, 1992). The Working Group asked the Information and Statistics Division of the NHS in Scotland (ISD Scotland) to report on the feasibility of producing a range of indicators on the basis of the national data sets of hospital discharge and death records.

> *The Clinical Outcomes Working Group is a subcommittee of the Clinical Resources and Audit Group (CRAG), a multi-disciplinary committee chaired by the Chief Medical Officer. CRAG is responsible to the Management Executive of the National Health Service in Scotland for the development of policies on clinical effectiveness issues including clinical audit, guidelines, outcomes and effective resource use.*

The foundations in terms of data were laid in 1967 when the commitment was made in Scotland that all hospital discharge records, cancer registrations and death records should be held centrally in machine-readable form with patient-identifying information such as name and date of birth to enable record linkage to take place. In 1988 a decision was made to move on from the previous ad hoc linkages and to create a permanently linked data set. By 1992 five years of data (1987–91) had been linked using probability matching (Kendrick and Clarke, 1993; Newcombe, 1988) and this linked data set provided a basis for five pilot measures to be produced for the working group. These were distributed within the Health Service at Health Board level in the summer of 1993 (Clinical Outcomes Working Group, 1993). Since then over thirty indicators have been published in four further reports (Clinical Outcomes Working Group, 1994; 1995; 1996; 1998) at Health Board, hospital or Trust level. The indicators are listed in Table 10.1.

General Features of the Indicators

Full details of the indicators are contained in the reports in which they are published. However, a few broad features should be outlined.

The published indicators cover a period of at least three years in order to minimize the role of random year on year variation. However, trend data on an annual basis have been distributed for some of the acute indicators and are always available to the relevant staff on request. Outcomes are only published

Table 10.1 Clinical outcome indicators reports 1993–98

Clinical outcome indicator	June 1993	Dec. 1994	Dec. 1995	July 1996	Mar. 1998
1 Teenage conception rate		B	B		
2 Therapeutic abortion rates		B	B		
3 Childhood incidence of measles		B			
4 Cervical cancer mortality		B	B		B
5 Suicide rate		B	B		
6 Rate of emergency admission for diabetic ketacidosis		B	B		
7 Longer inpatient stays for children with asthma		B	B		
8 30 day survival after admission for his fracture	B	T	T		
9 Discharge home within 56 days of admission with hip fracture	B	T	T		
10 30 day survival after admission for acute myocardial infarction	B	T	T		
11 Re-operation within 1 year of transurethral prostatectomy	B	T	T		
12 Medical specialties: emergency readmission within 28 days	B	T	T		
13 30 day survival after admission for stroke		T	T		
14 Discharge home within 56 days of admission for stroke		T	T		
15 Psychiatric inpatients: death within 1 year of discharge		H	H		
16 Psychiatric inpatients aged 65+: death within 1 year of discharge		H	H		
17 Psychiatric inpatients: suicide within 1 year of discharge		H	H		
18 Proportion of first births by caesarian section				H	
19 Vaginal delivery after caesarian section				H	
20 Babies admitted to a neonatal unit				H	
21 28 day emergency readmission: removal of tonsils/adenoids				T	
22 D & C rates				T	
23 Use of medical methods for early termination of pregnancy				B	
24 Survival with cancer of the trachea, bronchus and lung				B	
25 Survival with cancer of the large bowel				B	
26 Survival with breast cancer				B	
27 Survival with cancer of the ovary				B	
28 28 day emergency readmission: elective operation for cataract				T	
29 28 day emergency readmission: emergency appendectomy				T	
30 28 day emergency readmission: elective prostatectomy				T	
31 28 day emergency readmission: elective hysterectomy				T	
32 28 day emergency readmission: elective total hip replacement				T	
33 Survival with cancer of the stomach					B
34 Survival with cancer of the cervix uteri					B
35 Standardized procedure ratios for coronary angiography					B
36 Standardized procedure ratios for coronary angioplasty					B
37 Standardized procedure ratios for CABG					B
38 Standardized procedure ratios for angioplasty and CABG					B

Level of presentation: B = Health Board; T = Trust; H = Hospital.

for Trusts which have treated at least a minimum number of patients in the relevant category – usually 200 or 400 (cf. Hadorn et al., 1993). The indicators are standardized for whatever aspects of case mix are appropriate and can be derived from the available data. For example, the indicator of survival for 30 days after admission for heart attack is standardized for age, sex, small area deprivation score and any pre-existing conditions which have resulted in hospital admission.

Aims and Objectives

In the broadest sense, the initial aim of the production and publication of the indicators was to raise awareness in the NHS in Scotland of the importance of monitoring and comparing the outcomes of health care as a means to improving the quality of health care.

In the very first report, two rather more specific objectives were emphasized. The first was to highlight issues to do with the quality of the data on which the indicators are based. The second was that the identification of apparent variation in the outcome of treatment or health care in general between Trusts or Health Boards in Scotland would raise particular issues for discussion or further investigation (Clinical Outcomes Working Group, 1992).

It has been emphasized throughout the course of the production and publication of the indicators that they should not be regarded as direct measures of the quality of care provided. Wherever the indicators are reproduced the following warning accompanies them:

> It is stressed that no direct inferences about quality of care should be drawn from the indicators. They are intended rather to highlight issues which may require further investigation.

This recognition of the limitations of the indicators is a large part of the explanation of why their introduction in Scotland has taken place in a relatively uncontroversial and constructive manner.

Because they cannot provide proof in themselves about variation in quality of care the indicators are only useful when they are used by the Health Service as triggers for further enquiry or alongside other sources of insight. How the indicators were used and the effect they have had cannot be derived from a simple rational model of how the Health Service works but is highly dependent on the social and cultural make-up of the service and the beliefs and priorities of the actors involved as well as the wider political and cultural context. The reception given to the indicators provides some clues in this area.

Publication of the Indicators: The Response

The Context of Publication

We will look briefly at the response of several key constituencies: clinicians and management within the Health Service, the public and the media, and what might be called the health service research community in the widest sense. Crucial to a discussion of the response to the indicators is the simple fact that the indicators were published rather than circulated confidentially within the Health Service. Publication was not a foregone conclusion. The decision to publish the indicators, rather than use some method of distribution internal to the Health Service, was not taken lightly and only after intense discussion. Weighing against publication was the fear that it might lead to misuse and misinterpretation of the indicators resulting in potential distress to patients and professionals alike or to invalid decisions being taken. In favour of publication was the need to ensure a free flow of comparative information throughout the NHS in Scotland. Also in favour was a general presumption towards freedom of information and a desire to avoid a situation in which information relating to the quality of health care was being 'kept secret'. Perhaps the decisive factor was the acknowledgment that any system of circulating identifiable but not fully public outcomes information would inevitably lead to partial leaks and scare stories. Publication would allow proper contextualization of the information and explanation of the limitations of the indicators.

One particular aspect of the wider policy context had an immense impact on how the indicators were received by all the different audiences involved. This was a widespread 'league tables' agenda associated with a stress on competition and a particular emphasis on choice and accountability, especially in the area of education. It was inevitable that the publication of clinical outcome indicators in Scotland would be to some extent tarred with the league tables brush. This was a particular danger given the introduction of elements of the internal market and competition to the Health Service at the time. However, every effort was made to stress that the indicators were not league tables and should not be used as such. The indicators were not presented as rankings and even the relatively 'low tech', 'non-glossy' format of the reports was meant to convey the message that these were working documents rather than definitive assessments.

Clinicians and Managers

Responses to the indicators from clinicians and management within the Health Service varied immensely – from enthusiasm to hostility. Initially at least, it was apparent that managers were more favourable to the indicators than were clinicians.

Given that the indicators were in large part developed as a central initiative it was inevitable that there was almost no sense of ownership of the indicators and they were seen as being imposed from above. The fact that the indicators were published rather than being distributed internally also contributed to their being perceived as threatening.

One aspect of the reactions of those working in the NHS in Scotland is quite clear however. There has been virtually no simplistic and unquestioning use of the indicators to inform decisions without further enquiry. The indicators have not been used as league tables of quality within the National Health Service in Scotland. Despite fears to the contrary, no contracts were shifted on the basis of the indicators. It is equally clear that as the Health Service has become accustomed to the indicators, perceptions have in general shifted favourably so that they are increasingly seen as providing useful information.

The Public and the Media

Compared to what some had feared prior to publication, coverage of the indicators by the media has been on balance informed and responsible. The health correspondents of the Scottish press in particular provided in-depth and expert coverage. Although, as we have seen, every effort was made to stress that the indicators were not league tables, it was perhaps inevitable that the tabloids in particular would use this shorthand such as in the *Edinburgh Evening News*' somewhat ambiguous headline 'Capital Tops Death League Tables'.

The peak of interest in the broadcast media actually occurred before publication of the December 1994 report – the first published report to give outcomes at Trust level. In November 1994 when it became known that outcome indicators were to be published in Scotland there was a wave of interest by TV journalists on a UK level well as in Scotland, including talk shows, phone-in programmes, and political panel discussions. It was even reported in *The Independent* that the Cabinet was split over whether the precocious Scots should be allowed to proceed (*The Independent*, 1994).

The actual publication of the December 1994 report led to some UK press coverage and the highest level of Scottish coverage – including a good deal at local level. After the 1994 report however, the only coverage at the UK level has been in specialist medical journals, or as context to any proposals to produce outcome indicators in England and Wales. The second report (December 1995 – published February 1996) produced a day of Scottish press, TV and radio coverage. More recent reports produced a somewhat lower level of Scottish coverage. Coverage in the local press continues to be alert to any apparently poor outcomes on the part of the local Health Board or hospital. However, the hope is largely being fulfilled that the indicators will cease to be a major news item and will increasingly become part of the routine circulation of information in the Health Service.

Most importantly however, there was very little evidence that publication of the indicators produced public unease or distress. There were isolated instances of individuals being worried about the quality of care being received by relatives, but the Scottish Association of Health Councils, for example, reported almost no enquiries on the part of the public. So successful in fact was the promulgation of the message that no immediate implications should be drawn from the indicators that the press has been almost as inclined to complain about the cost and usefulness of the indicators as it has been to trumpet any scandal about variations in the quality of care. There is a very fine line to be trodden in how such indicators are presented.

The Health Service Research Community

In many ways the most consistently negative responses tended to emanate from the medical and health service research community. Many articles were directed towards the English policy context and were overwhelmingly concerned to point out the dangers of drawing premature implications about quality of care and to point out that the dangers of publication outweighed the benefits (Orchard, 1994; McKee and Hunter, 1995; Davies, 1997). This largely negative response can perhaps best be understood in terms of two factors: the previously mentioned league tables agenda and the fact that most contributions formed part of a discourse defined in terms of statistical proof and disproof. Whether this is the most productive framework for debate is discussed below.

Impact of the Indicators: Results of a Survey

In June 1997 62 questionnaires were issued by the CRAG Secretariat to the

Medical Directors of all 47 Trusts and to the Directors of Public Health at the 15 Health Boards in Scotland. After two reminder letters, 61 forms (98 per cent) were returned. The stated purpose of the survey was: '*To obtain a comprehensive picture of the use made of the outcome indicators published by the Clinical Outcomes Working Group of CRAG*'. To facilitate analysis, Trusts and Health Boards were asked to record their responses according to one of seven categories, A–F or not applicable. Responses to the 31 indicators from 47 Trusts and 15 Health Boards meant that there were 1,922 responses in total. Table 10.2 below summarizes the responses.

Table 10.2   Responses to survey on impact of outcome indicators

	Response	No.	%
A	The indicator was not seen by the relevant clinicians	57	3.0
B	The indicator was not useful at all	207	10.8
C	The indicator was of interest but did not raise any issue of concern to my hospital/specialty/Trust/Health Board	738	38.4
D	The indicator raised an issue of concern which led to discussion but no further action	162	8.4
E	The indicator raised an issue of concern which led to further investigation (such as data analysis, audit review, special data collection, etc.) but no change in practice	119	6.2
F	The indicator raised an issue of concern which brought about, or helped to bring about a change to the service (such as a change in working patterns or clinical practice, allocation of additional resources or new facilities)	78	4.1
No response	Indicator not applicable, or response not completed	530	27.6
No reply	Trust did not complete survey	31	1.6
Total		1,922	100.0

Given that the indicators include some which are relevant to only a narrow selection of Trusts (e.g. the psychiatric or maternity indicators) and some Trusts cater for only a narrow clientele (e.g. children's hospitals, the dental hospital), the high number of responses which were not applicable, or left blank ('No response') is not altogether surprising.

The single most common response was C – indicating that 'the indicator was of interest but did not raise any issue of concern to my hospital/specialty/Trust/Health Board'. This was expected, given that for most indicators the majority of organizations are close to the Scottish mean.

Overall, the findings of the survey suggest that the indicators generated a considerable amount of discussion, some additional clinical audit and, less often but most importantly, changes to practice. In nearly 200 instances it was reported that an indicator led to further investigation, or helped to bring about a change to the service (that is, responses E and F). Notably, in the indicators which had the greatest impact, a majority of those with results significantly below the Scottish mean reported that they had taken some action. It is not claimed that the indicators were the sole cause of this activity, but that publication of the indicators was a useful catalyst.

With a few exceptions such as the establishment of several stroke units, (and here one comment is telling – 'The indicator provided additional information to support the case for establishing an Acute Stroke Unit'), the actions reported as being taken following publication were by and large modest rather than dramatic – audits undertaken, working practices amended, guidelines implemented, research initiated. Such results certainly lack the drama of contracts being shifted, but given the limitations of currently available outcome indicators, it is surely a measure of success that the indicators were of practical value.

Evidence into Action: The Logic

The practical path by which information on outcomes can be translated into information about quality of care, and can thus provide a basis for improving the quality of care, has been given many expressions.

The recent NHS Executive Consultation Document on assessing performance in the NHS in England contains a concise formulation when it states that the new framework for performance assessment 'will encourage greater benchmarking of performance in different areas, and the publication of comparative information will allow people to compare performance and share best practice' (NHS Executive, 1998).

When accounts of the classic audit feedback loop contain reference to outcomes a similar logic is involved (Lakhani, 1995).

A specification of the full path of implication might contain the following elements:

1   an outcome indicator highlights possible suboptimal performance;

2   further investigation confirms that the variation in the indicator reflects a real difference in the quality of care;

3   further investigation is able to attribute the difference in quality of care to identifiable differences in the way health care is provided: whether the differences lie in the resources available, the method of treatment, or the efficiency with which treatment is delivered;

4   action is taken to remedy the deficiency in provision of care.

Even this basic formulation represents a long and vulnerable chain of implications and actions to be expected of the staff of the Health Service. The lesson of the survey reported in the previous section is that the improvements made on the basis of the indicators rarely reflected an explicit implementation of this full logic. It should also be noted such a model does not require the indicators in themselves to provide proof of variation in the quality of care.

Lessons Learned and Ways Forward: Influences on the Constructive Use of Outcome Indicators

In this section we outline some of the factors which appear to have influenced the extent to which the clinical outcome indicators published in Scotland helped improve care. These factors divide broadly into those to do with the nature and presentation of the indicators themselves, and those to do with how they have been received and used by the Health Service. Discussion of these issues leads naturally into some thoughts on how the monitoring of outcomes might best be carried forward.

A   Production and Presentation of the Indicators

The validity of the indicators The general issue of the extent to which outcome indicators can act as valid pointers to variation in the quality of care has received a great deal of methodological attention. The classic account is now over 10 years old (Blumberg, 1986) and an extensive literature has accumulated since, especially in the United States (e.g. Krakauer et al., 1992; Hadorn et al., 1993).

Our interest is practical. Unless the outcome indicator bears a reasonably straightforward relationship to the desired outcome of care, both in principle and assuming all data issues of accuracy and case mix have been overcome, then it is useless and will be quite rightly ignored or resented. The Scottish outcome indicators have varied in the extent to which they have met this criterion. Among the best indicators have been some of those relating to survival. The survival of the patient can usually be taken as the objective of care although even here there are issues, especially when palliative care is involved. (An indicator of survival after surgery for colo-rectal cancer was dropped at an early stage because it would have been impossible to take account of palliative aspects.) However, the indicators which showed various aspects of mortality after discharge from psychiatric inpatient care have received considerable unfavourable comment since it is very difficult to attribute these outcomes to the process of care involved. Similarly, it has been shown that fewer than half of emergency readmissions after cataract surgery are clinically related to the procedure (Purdie and Jay, 1998; Cox and Simpson, 1998).

The quality of the data The data sources upon which the indicators are based have a high reputation when compared with similar data elsewhere (Brewster et al., 1996; Harley and Jones, 1996). The accuracy of the linkage of these records to each other and to Registrar General's death records is at least 99 per cent (Kendrick and Clarke, 1993). However, the SMR1 hospital discharge records in particular were designed over 30 years ago and were not constructed as a basis for outcome indicators. The key parameter of accuracy is that coding of principal diagnosis at the ICD9 three-digit level is around 90 per cent accurate with no evidence of systematic bias (Clinical Outcomes Working Group, 1995).

The more it is felt that any variation in apparent outcome can be attributed to the inadequacies of the data, the less incentive there is to carry out any further investigation to confirm the variation or otherwise. The first response to any apparent negative outcome is often to question the accuracy of the data. However, apart from highly specific exceptions attributable to local breakdowns of coding procedures, in all the dozens of occasions when Trusts or Health Boards have asked ISD Scotland to check the validity of the data involved, further investigation has confirmed its essential.

The role of case mix variation Even where the quality of the data coding is satisfactory in terms of the transfer of information from the case notes or discharge letter to the coded central returns, there remains a more fundamental issue. Broadly speaking, variation in outcome may reflect variation in the characteristics (case mix) of the patients, or variation in quality of the care provided. The data available in Scotland has permitted standardization (where appropriate) for such factors as age, sex, a small-area based deprivation index and pre-existing morbidity as indicated by previous admissions to hospital.

We do not have a direct measure of the severity of patients' conditions on admission. It is this feature of the indicators which has been perhaps the major focus of criticism of their validity (Davenport et al., 1997).

In the case of 30-day survival after admission for heart attack, as for the indicators of acute care in general, standardization for deprivation and pre-existing morbidity made very little difference at hospital level (Capewell et al., 1996). This would suggest that it is unlikely that variation in case mix independent of these factors would play a great role. However, we still have no solid empirical evidence either way about the role of variation in patient severity independent of the factors for which we have been able to standardize in accounting for variation in outcome.

The timeliness of the data One deficiency in the data which has acted as a barrier to the constructive use of the outcome indicators is that the indicators have always been at least a year out-of-date due to the cycle of data processing and linkage. Again, this reduces the incentive to follow-up any variations.

Presentation and analysis As is stressed repeatedly wherever the outcome indicators are reproduced, the objective is not to provide immediate proof. The indicators in themselves are not intended to provide proof that the quality of care in one institution is better than in another. They can provide evidence which can usually only become proof when used in conjunction with other more sensitive local or comparative information. In this context it is interesting that where action has been taken which has been influenced by the outcome indicators, it is often where the indicators confirm a suspicion which has been formed on other grounds.

The success with which this message can be got across when the information is presented is limited by the statistical language which we have available for presenting the indicators. The language of statistics is still dominated by the language of proof and disproof. The aim of statistics as a discipline has largely been to provide techniques to turn the messiness of real events into numbers which can provide black and white, yes/no answers to specific questions. This is perhaps especially true of medical statistics where the overriding aim is often to prove whether or not a treatment is effective.

When it was decided that the indicators should be provided with confidence intervals, this was done in part so that small differences in apparent outcome should not be over-interpreted as demonstrating a difference in the quality of care. However, the introduction of confidence intervals may have had the perverse effect of inviting readers to interpret the indicators according to the statistical language of proof (or significance testing), i.e. it is only worth taking account of a variation from the Scottish mean if the Scottish mean falls outwith the confidence interval for a given Trust.

The actual contribution of the academic statistical community to the outcome indicators debate has tended to mire it ever deeper in this inappropriate emphasis on proof rather than evidence. Particularly unhelpful here has been discussion of outcome indicators in terms of league tables and rankings (Goldstein and Spiegelhalter, 1996; Leyland and Boddy, 1998; Parry et al., 1998). As already mentioned, the Health Service in Scotland has thankfully remained immune to treating the indicators as league tables and discussion of Health Service outcomes in terms of rankings is patently inappropriate (Hannan, 1998).

It has been suggested that greater use should be made of more sophisticated methods of statistical modelling, and in particular multi-level modelling in the analysis and case-mix adjustment of outcome indicators (Goldstein and Spiegelhalter, 1996; Nutley and Smith, 1998). Although any contribution which helps control for confounding factors is welcome, we must sound a cautionary note here. We have been very clear in Scotland about the limitations of the data on which the indicators are based. There is a danger that the application of ever more sophisticated techniques will add more to the illusion than to the actuality that definitive conclusions can be drawn from the indicators.

There is also an issue of clarity. Clinicians are the key audience for outcome indicators. There are, of course, other audiences – planners, patients and policy makers – but unless indicators are judged as credible and legitimate by 'ordinary clinicians', they will have little currency for other groups. Credibility requires indicators to be meaningful and understandable to those who are expected to make use of them. Adjustments to indicators, therefore, need to be kept as transparent as possible. Further investigations, and the addition of information from other sources, should be the way to answer any questions raised by the indicators, rather than subjecting the data to pre-publication 'analysis' and complex multivariate modelling. This may only serve to render the indicators mysterious and incomprehensible and deprive them of credibility. It was decided at an early stage to keep the Scottish indicators as free from statistical jargon and formulae as possible and to use well understood methods such as standardization as far as possible.

B   The Use Made of the Indicators

It is becoming a commonplace of other areas of evidence-based medicine that the mere provision of evidence (whether in the form of published research, Cochrane reviews or even explicit guidelines and protocols) does not lead directly towards change in practice (Grimshaw and Russell, 1993 and 1994). Much of this work echoes an earlier and classic statement of the lack of impact of long-standing evidence on variation in practice (Evans, 1990). Rather, the translation of the provision of evidence into change in the practice of health care is a process which is mediated by the immensely complex social, professional, organizational and cultural system which is the health care delivery system (Lomas, 1993). To quote the opening words of a recent editorial in *Quality in Health Care*:

> An accepted approach to seeking to change clinical practice assumes a fairly straightforward relation between clinical evidence, the development and publication of national guidelines, the acknowledgement of national guidelines in local protocols, and the day-to-day behaviour of clinicians. The notion that we can understand these relations in terms of a single input-output linear model is considerably challenged by any work which examines any part of this assumed process (Dawson, 1997).

In other words, even when there is overwhelming evidence of the best way of doing things, evidence endorsed by the panoply of national guidance and guidelines, it cannot be taken for granted that the desired change in behaviour will take place.

Outcome indicators are not about overwhelming evidence. They are about clues and suggestions that there may in certain places be better ways of doing things. They are about helping to find out what these better ways might be and putting them into practice. Outcome indicators are concerned with a wider range of factors than other forms of evidence-based practice in that they are not simply concerned with which methods of treatment are the best but with the entire set of inputs to the treatment process. This would suggest that taking action on the basis of outcome indicators is a much more fragile and complex process than any of those involved in translating more explicit forms of evidence into practice.

This makes it all the more important to address the question of whether the National Health Service in Scotland has had the knowledge and skills, the time and resources and the motivation and supportive culture to make best use of the clinical outcome indicators.

These issues of social and cultural context are all the more important in that the indicators concern extremely sensitive, literally life and death, issues relating to the quality of care. They impinge on the self-esteem and the professional reputation of clinicians. Like other areas of evidence-based medicine they raise issues of clinical freedom and the individualistic nature of medical decision-making. They raise issues of managerial versus clinical areas of control and influence. Such issues were compounded in the early 1990s when the NHS in Scotland seemed to be moving towards an internal market and more competitive mechanisms.

One of the most fundamental considerations is that Scotland is the only country in the world currently publishing national clinical outcome indicators at hospital level. Other countries, and in particular the United States, have built up considerable experience over the last decade in the production, analysis and theory of outcome indicators but relatively little material is available about how they can best be used on the ground to influence the day-to-day running of the health service. In other words, there were almost no precedents available for the clinical staff who were expected to make sense of and make use of the indicators.

Even if we can foster the right technical, organizational and interpersonal skills and engineer a much greater knowledge of the outcomes perspective throughout the Health Service, it will count for little without further development of an organizational culture within the Health Service which is more supportive to the constructive use of outcome indicators.

By and large, the culture of the Health Service is not one that is attuned to the kind of activity which is called for in order to make maximum use of the evidence which outcome indicators provide. If change is to be achieved by consensual rather than coercive means, two models in particular offer concrete pointers.

The first is clinical audit. Audit has been called a 'secret garden' and the significant expenditure on it over the last decade has been criticized because it has not been seen to deliver the promised impact on practice. However, what clinical audit can achieve in the best circumstances is the kind of exchange of information about outcomes and how things are done which can improve practice. Here defensiveness is overcome in a context of confidentiality and mutual professional trust. It is likely that some of the most constructive discussion of the comparative implications of the Scottish outcome indicators has taken place in the context of audit networks.

The other model which offers a way forward is the benchmarking club. Benchmarking developed as a highly commonsensical procedure. Given a competitive environment in which several companies are carrying out similar activities, how does a company find out the best way to perform said activity? One way is to compare the various companies on a range of reasonable indicators of performance, find out who is performing best on the basis of the indicators and find out how they do it. In the Health Service, more collaborative implementation in the form of the benchmarking club, as has been piloted in terms of groupings of Trusts in Scotland, is perhaps more appropriate.

Where clinical audit and benchmarking have succeeded in practical terms in using the sharing of comparative information to move towards best practice they have done so by creating structures for discussion which remove defensiveness and foster the open exchange of practical experience. They have created protective micro-environments in which trust exists and in which fruitful discussion and investigation can take place.

The challenge for the Health Service is to create similar structures at a more general level: to create a culture of comparison in which comparative information is to be welcomed as an opportunity for learning rather than feared (Hunter, 1998). Outcomes information has been proposed as a key element in moving towards the 'learning hospital' (Pfaff, 1995). National outcome indicators will only come into their own to the extent that we move towards a 'learning Health Service'.

At a more immediate level, many of the practical steps which we can take to make the clinical outcome indicators more effective will take us closer to best practice in clinical audit as exemplified by some of the national comparative audits now coming to maturity in Scotland such as the Scottish Trauma Audit Group and the National Hip Fracture Audit.

First of all, the outcome information must be much more up-to-date. Current redevelopment of the national data sets and record linkage methodology means that it will be possible to feed back national outcome information within a few months rather than having to wait over a year. More flexible and routine ways of distributing the information to the Health Service will need to be developed.

Another way forward will involve the development of ways of incorporating much more sensitive condition specific and specialty specific outcomes related information into routine data sources. In particular this will allow outcomes monitoring to adjust for case-mix in a more satisfactory manner. The addition of condition-specific items on severity of condition and related process measures is currently being piloted in Scotland.

Such exercises require much closer involvement by the relevant groups of specialist clinicians. This in turn is perhaps the most important area in which the production of clinical outcome information needs to move towards the best practice of clinical audit.

As the outcomes perspective continues to spread throughout Health Service practice, it is altogether possible that the current clear distinction between clinical outcome indicators developed and produced at the centre and audit programmes set up and run by clinicians and other professional groups will begin to break down. Whether outcomes are monitored as national indicators or as part of comparative audit will be a purely pragmatic question: which works best?

Conclusions

In terms of two of the relatively limited aims set out at the beginning of the enterprise – the highlighting of issues to do with the quality of the data on which the indicators are based and the raising of the general level of awareness of the outcomes perspective – the publication of clinical outcomes indicators in Scotland has fulfilled its remit.

In terms of the more ambitious objective of actually making a difference to the quality of health care in Scotland by raising appropriate questions about specific variations in quality of care the indicators have, as we have seen, had an effect but there is a long way to go. This chapter has been largely about existing barriers to making the most effective use of outcome indicators. An important message is that outcome indicators do not have to be perfect to be useful (Hannan, 1998).

Much of the abstract academic discussion of outcome indicators over the past few years has suggested that it is irresponsible and dangerous to produce and, even more so, to publish clinical outcome indicators unless these indicators in themselves can provide absolute proof of specific variations in quality of care. Our perspective is quite different. Currently available data cannot support the kind of proof of variation in quality of care which is often demanded. All that indicators based on such data can do is open up issues for further investigation. Thereafter there may a be wide range of appropriate and constructive responses ranging from immediate and common sense incremental improvements to larger scale changes in service provision. We can however suggest that the more any follow-up to the indicators is collaborative and comparative, the more likely it is to make full use of whatever evidence and clues the indicators might furnish as to where best-practice might be lacking and to where best-practice might be found. This however makes great demands on the Health Service.

Until now, in Scotland and elsewhere, the vast bulk of the effort devoted to clinical outcome indicators has been channelled into the technical process of the production of the indicators: ensuring that they are valid, meaningful and well presented. In other words the emphasis has been on the production of the indicators.

It is becoming ever more clear at a Scottish level, at a UK level (McColl et al., 1996) and more generally (Nutley and Smith, 1998) that just as much emphasis needs to be placed on understanding how outcome indicators can best be used.

The current culture and organization of the National Health Service is not geared to making the most effective use of the information about the outcome of care which is available to it. Outcome indicators in Scotland were delivered to a Service which by and large, with significant exceptions, was not sure what to do with them. Publication certainly ensured that the indicators were taken seriously but the only other driving forces were exhortation and the implicit commitment of the NHS to delivering high quality health care.

However the events and policy developments of 1998 look set to change this picture utterly. The Bristol tragedy has focused the minds of everyone on the importance of monitoring outcomes and, crucially, of taking action when they provide grounds for concern that quality is bad. There are signs that the required cultural shift is beginning.

This will be massively reinforced by the various policy initiatives north and south of the border aimed at making improvement in the quality of care the explicit rather than merely the implicit driver of the National Health Service (Scottish Office Department of Health, 1997 and 1998; Department of Health 1998). In particular, clinical governance will give a statutory basis to NHS Trusts' responsibility for quality.

Clinical outcomes indicators will have a key role to play in the new framework. In turn the new initiatives aimed at clinical quality will help provide the cultural context and organizational structures which are necessary to make the best use of information on the outcomes of care.

Clinical outcome indicators are tools to be used rather than clubs to be wielded. The new framework should bring us closer to realizing the promise of constructive and committed use of these tools for quality.[1]

Note

1   The authors would like to acknowledge in particular Mrs Eileen Barnwell and Dr Dorothy Moir who have done more than anyone to push forward the clinical outcomes agenda in Scotland. For helpful comments on this paper we would like to thank Jim Chalmers, Richard

Copland, Roger Black, David Brewster, Marion Bain, Andrew Fraser, Willie Farquhar and David Steel. The views expressed however are the responsibility of the authors alone.

References

Blumberg, M.S. (1986), 'Risk Adjusting Health Care Outcomes: A methodologic review', *Medical Care Review*, 43, pp. 351–93.

Brewster, D., Crichton, J. and Muir, C.S. (1996), 'How Accurate are Scottish Cancer Registration Data?', *British Journal of Cancer*, 70, pp. 954–9.

Capewell, S., Kendrick, S., Boyd, S., Cohen, G., Juszczak, E. and Clarke, J. (1996), 'Measuring Outcomes: One month survival after acute myocardial infarction in Scotland', *Heart*, 76, pp. 70–5.

Clinical Outcomes Working Group (1992), *Clinical Outcome Measures: an interim report by a Working Group set up by the Management Executive*, Clinical Resource and Audit Group, The Scottish Office, NHS in Scotland.

Clinical Outcomes Working Group (1993), *Clinical Outcome Measures Report, June 1993*, Clinical Resource and Audit Group, The Scottish Office, NHS in Scotland.

Clinical Outcomes Working Group (1994), *Clinical Outcome Indicators Report, December 1994*, Clinical Resource and Audit Group, The Scottish Office, NHS in Scotland.

Clinical Outcomes Working Group (1995), *Clinical Outcome Indicators Report, December 1995*, Clinical Resource and Audit Group, The Scottish Office, NHS in Scotland.

Clinical Outcomes Working Group (1996), *Clinical Outcome Indicators Report, July 1996*, Clinical Resource and Audit Group, The Scottish Office, NHS in Scotland.

Clinical Outcomes Working Group (1998), *Clinical Outcome Indicators Report, March 1998*, Clinical Resource and Audit Group, The Scottish Office, NHS in Scotland.

Clinical Resource and Audit Group (1989), *Health Care Outcome Indicators*, report from a Working Group.

Cox, A. and Simpson, W.A.C. (1998), 'The Use of Readmission Rates as a Measure of Clinical Outcome Following Cataract Surgery', *Health Bulletin (Edinburgh)*, 56, pp. 799–802.

Davies, H. (1997), 'What's a healthy outcome?', *Health Service Journal*, 10 April, p. 22.

Dawson, S. (1997), 'Inhabiting Different Worlds: How can research relate to practice', *Quality in Health Care*, 6, pp. 177–8.

Department of Health (1998), *A First Class Service: Quality in the new NHS*.

Evans, R.G. (1990), 'The Dog in the Night-time: Medical Practice Variations and Health Policy' in T.F. Anderson and G. Mooney (eds), *The Challenges of Medical Practice Variations*, Macmillan, Basingstoke.

Goldstein, H. and Spiegelhalter, D.J. (1996), 'League Tables and their Limitations: Statistical Issues in Comparisons of Institutional Performance', *Journal of the Royal Statistical Society, Series A*, 159 Part 3.

Grimshaw, J.M. and Russell, I.T. (1993), 'Effects of Clinical Guidelines on Medical Practice. A Systematic Review of Rigorous Evaluations', *Lancet*, 342, pp. 1317–22.

Grimshaw, J.M. and Russell, I.T. (1994), 'Achieving Health Gain Through Clinical Guidelines II: Ensuring guidelines change medical practice', *Quality in Health Care*, 3 (1), pp. 45–52.

Hadorn, D.C., Keeler, E.B., Rogers, W.H. and Brook, R.H. (1993), *Assessing the Performance of Mortality Prediction Models*, RAND/UCLA/Harvard Center for Health Care Financing Policy Research.

Hannan, E.H. (1998), 'Measuring Hospital Outcomes: Don't make perfect the enemy of the good!', *Journal of Health Service Research and Policy*, 3, pp. 67–9.

Harley, K. and Jones, C. (1996), 'Quality of Scottish Morbidity Record (SMR) data', *Health Bulletin (Edinburgh)*, 54, pp. 410–7.

Hunter, D. (1998), 'A case of under-management', *Health Service Journal*, 25 June, pp. 18–19.

Kendrick, S. and Clarke, J. (1993), 'The Scottish Record Linkage System', *Health Bulletin*, 51 (2), pp. 72–9.

Krakauer, H., Bailey, R.C., Skellan, K.J., Stewart, J.D., Hartz, A.J., Kuhn, E.M. and Rimm, A.R. (1992), 'Evaluation of the HCFA Model for the Analysis of Mortality Following Hospitalisation', *Health Services Research*, 27 (3), pp. 318–35.

Lakhani, A. (1995), 'The Role of Outcomes Assessment in Improving Clinical Effectiveness in M. Deighan and S. Hitch (eds), *Clinical Effectiveness from Guidelines to Cost-Effective Practice*, Earlybrave Publications Ltd, Brentwood.

Leyland, A. and Boddy, F.A. (1998), 'League Tables and Acute Myocardial Infarction', *The Lancet*, 351, pp. 555–8.

Lomas, J. (1993), *Teaching Old (and Not so Old) Docs New Tricks: Effective ways to implement research findings*, CHEPA Working Paper Series No. 93–4 April, McMaster University, Hamilton, Ontario.

McColl, A., Ferris, G., Roderick, P. and Gabbay, J. (1996), *How do English DHAs use Population Health Outcome Assessments?*, University of Southampton.

McKee, M. and Hunter, D. (1995), 'Mortality League Tables: Do they inform or mislead?', *Quality in Health Care*, 4 (1), pp. 5–12.

Newcombe, H. (1988), *Handbook of record linkage*, Oxford University Press, New York.

NHS Executive (1998), *The New NHS, Modern and Dependable: A National Framework for Assessing Performance*, NHS Executive Consultation Document.

Nutley, S. and Smith, P.C. (1998), 'League Tables for Performance Improvement in Health Care', *Journal of Health Services Research and Policy*, 3 (1), pp. 50–7.

Orchard, C. (1994), 'Comparing healthcare outcomes', *British Medical Journal*, 308, pp. 1493–6.

Parry G.J., Gould, C.R., McCabe, C.J. and Tarnow-Mordi, W.O. (1998), 'Annual League Tables of Mortality in Neonatal Intensive Care Units: Longitudinal study', *British Medical Journal*, 310, pp. 1931–5.

Pfaff, H. (1995), 'Managing for Health Outcomes as a Central Element of the 'Learning Hospital': Concept, Methodologues, Problems', paper for EHMA Annual Scientific Meeting, Celle, Germany.

Purdie, A.T. and Jay, J.L. (1998), 'Interpretation of Statistics for Emergency Readmissions Following Cataract Surgery', *Health Bulletin (Edinburgh)*, 56, pp. 641–4.

Scottish Office Department of Health (1997), *Designed to Care: Renewing the National Health Service in Scotland*, The Stationery Office, Edinburgh.

Scottish Office Department of Health (1998), *Acute Services Review Report*, The Stationery Office, Edinburgh.

The Independent (1994), 21 November.

11 What do Managers and Physicians Prefer as Indicators of Clinical Outcome?

RÉGIS BLAIS,[1, 2] DANIELLE LAROUCHE,[1] PIERRE BOYLE,[3] RAYNALD PINEAULT [1, 3] AND SERGE DUBÉ[4]

1   Groupe de recherche interdisciplinaire en santé, Faculté de médecine, Université de Montréal
2   Département d'administration de la santé, Faculté de médecine, Université de Montréal
3   Département de médecine sociale et préventive, Faculté de médecine, Université de Montréal
4   Département de chirurgie, Hôpital Maisonneuve-Rosemont

Context

Organizational performance assessment is essential to maintain and improve quality of health care services (Leggat et al., 1998). There is not, however a single accepted and adopted model (Sicotte et al., 1998), although performance indicators have been developed and evaluated for a number of years (Leggat et al., 1998). One type of indicator considered as an instrument to assess the quality of care is clinical outcome indicators. Studies documenting clinical outcomes of different types of health care interventions have multiplied in the last two decades (Mitchell et al., 1997). The results of these studies, when combined with other types of information, can be very useful to physicians with administrative responsibilities and hospital managers in their efforts to change aspects of the organization and delivery of the services in order to improve the quality of health care.

The popularity of the concept of evidence-based medicine attests to a need for the use of scientific data in the decision-making process (Klein, 1996; Maynard, 1997). There are many examples of feedback and benchmarking programmes that have influenced surgical rates (Dyck et al., 1977; Wennberg

Managing Quality: Strategic Issues in Health Care Management, H.T.O. Davies, M. Tavakoli, M. Malek, A.R. Neilson (eds), Ashgate Publishing Ltd, 1999.

173

et al., 1977) and led to shorter hospital lengths of stay (Billi et al., 1992; Manheim et al., 1990) or to a decrease in drug prescription (Kroenke et al., 1990). Hospital report cards have been shown to help improve hospital quality of care (Rainwater et al., 1998). In spite of the development of many new tools, hospital physicians and managers seem to find it difficult to use the results of the studies.

There are probably many explanations for these difficulties, the main one being that the type of information available is not adapted to the individual needs of potential users (Lomas, 1997). Certain information may be lacking. For example, the information might not include enough detail to be useful for decision-making, the data used might not be recent enough or the information might not be presented in an appealing way. Despite numerous studies concerning the diffusion of information in the health field (e.g. Grady et al., 1993), we know very little about what managers and physicians with administrative responsibilities deem useful as indicators of clinical outcomes. To maximize the usefulness of information on health services results, it is not enough to generate data; it is also essential to know what content and form of presentation would facilitate their effective use by managers and physicians with administrative responsibilities in the field. In other words, to be able to make sound decisions, clinicians, managers and policy makers need to have access to information that they understand and are able to use (Flood et al., 1994).

Our research project, currently under way, attempts to answer some of those questions, using an interactive approach in which the content and presentation of postsurgical complications indicators are progressively adjusted to meet the needs of hospital managers and physicians in the province of Quebec, Canada.

The objectives of our project are:

1 to identify the type of content and form of presentation of clinical outcome measures that managers and physicians with administrative responsibilities consider useful. The study focuses on postsurgical complications of three frequent interventions (cholecystectomy, hysterectomy and prostatectomy). These interventions serve as tracers or examples;

2 to identify user and hospital characteristics associated with differences expressed by managers and physicians as to the content and form of presentation of those clinical outcome measures;

3 to measure managers' and physicians' actual utilization of the outcome measures and identify factors that facilitate or prevent their use, as well as solutions to overcome the obstacles encountered.

The research activities of this project are organized in eight steps, alternating between consultations with experts and potential users of data and the production and analysis of data by the research team (Figure 11.1). The first step, which is the subject of this paper, consisted of two meetings during which we consulted with managers and physicians.

The opinions expressed during these consultations will be used as the basis for postsurgical complications reports sent to 30 selected hospitals (step 2). These reports will be sent to eight to 10 key managers or physicians who have responsibilities in evaluating the care given in their hospital (step 3).

With the report, each person will receive a questionnaire for evaluating the usefulness of the content and the appropriateness of the presentation of the report (step 4). This first survey will enable us to adapt a second report that will be prepared with more recent data (step 5) and identify user and hospital characteristics associated with differences expressed by managers and physicians (step 6). The second report will be followed by a second survey, to measure managers' and physicians' actual utilization of the reports and identify factors that facilitated or prevented their use (step 7). The last step (step 8) will consist of analysing the data and writing the final research report.

The object of this chapter is to present the methods and results from the first step, i.e., the consultations with experts.

Objective and Methods

The objective of the initial consultations was to gather information from current or potential users of hospital clinical outcome measures on the nature and format of presentation of postsurgical complication data that would be useful to them. To be able to distinguish between the needs and preferences of managers and those of physicians with administrative responsibilities, we held two separate sessions.

Seven managers and seven physicians were identified and selected for their expertise and willingness to participate. Since statistical represent-ativeness was not an objective, the participants were chosen based on their experience with and interest in the utilization of clinical outcome measures to improve the quality of health care. The participants came from university and

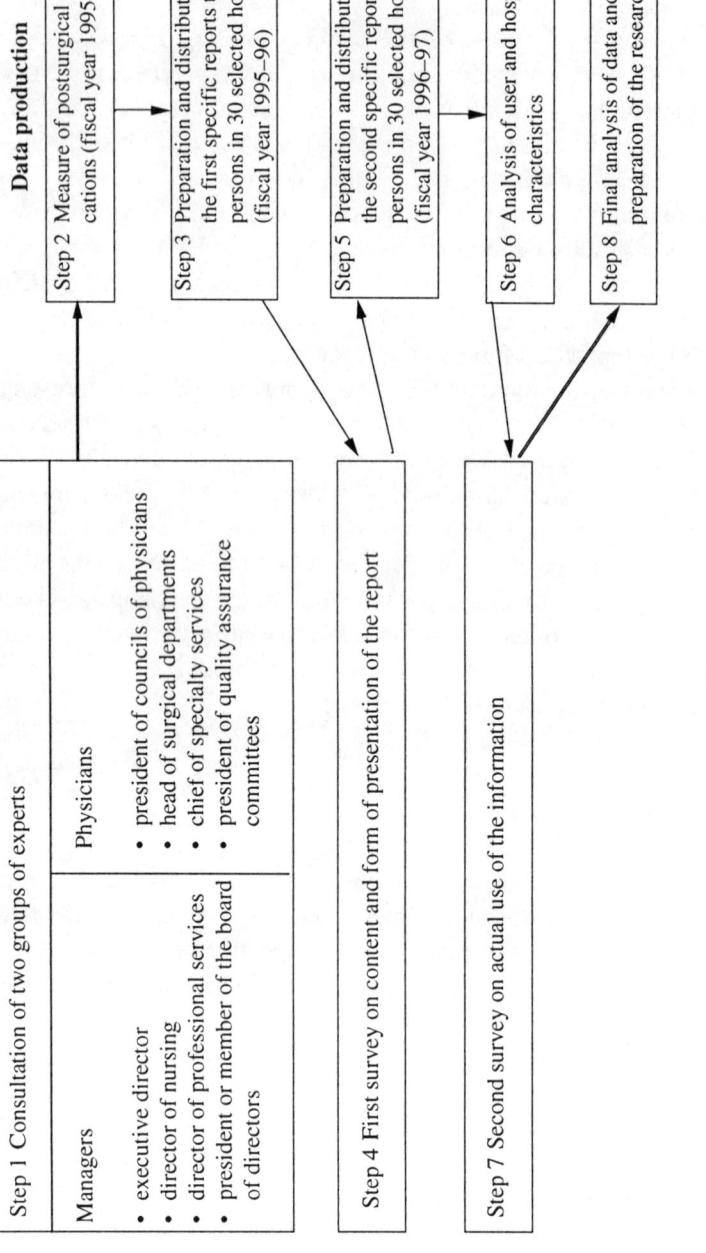

Figure 11.1 Steps in the research project

non-university affiliated acute care hospitals in the metropolitan Montreal area. The group of managers consisted of members of boards of directors of acute care hospitals, executive directors, and directors of both nursing and professional services. Physicians with administrative responsibilities were represented by presidents of medical councils, heads of surgical departments, chiefs of specialty services, and presidents of hospital quality assurance committees.

A modified nominal group technique (Delbecq and Van de Ven, 1971) was used for both meetings, which each lasted a little over two hours. The meetings started with a short presentation of the objectives and methodology of the project by members of the research team. The objectives of the meeting and the four themes to be discussed were then explained to the participants: the content of outcome reports, their presentation, the characteristics of the information to be included, and the type of surgical procedures to be prioritized. The participants were informed that the research project focused on postsurgical complications, but the indicators that we hoped to develop were not mentioned to them so that their opinions would not be influenced by this information.

During the meetings, one member of the research team served as moderator while another wrote items on a board. For each of the four themes, the nominal group process went as follows. First, each participant presented in turn his or her ideas and suggestions without comment from the others. All items were written on the board for everyone to see. Second, a period of clarification and discussion of the items followed; similar items could then be combined and new ones could be added. Third, the participants wrote down their top priority items (up to 10) on prepared voting forms. Fourth, forms were collected and, to maximize the time spent on discussion, the votes were tallied after the meeting. Votes were weighted according to the ranks of the items (e.g. on a list of 10 items, the item ranked number 1 was given a weight of 10, the item ranked number 2 a weight of 9, etc.) As a courtesy to the participants, the results of the vote were sent to them afterwards by mail.

Results

Tables 11.1–11.3 present the results of the consultations with the group of managers and the group of physicians for three of the four themes discussed. Results of the fourth theme are described in the text only. Items in tables are listed in descending order of priority according to the votes (score). Items receiving fewer than seven points (i.e. less than one point per participant on average) were excluded.

Table 11.1 presents the elements that managers and physicians would like to find in reports on surgical outcomes. An important distinction has to be made between two types of items listed by the participants. The first type concerns indicators of complications as such (items 2, 9,10 and 15). It is interesting to note that two of those indicators were already considered for development by the research team (complications during the hospitalization and rehospitalization for complications). The second type groups items that serve as stratification variables. These variables allow the examination of the performance indicators from different angles (e.g. type of surgery, level of case severity).

Both groups would like detailed information, but the physicians' preferences included a larger number of items. Eleven of the 16 items on the managers' list are also present on the physicians' list, but they do not have the same priority. Yet of the five top priorities for each group, three are the same, i.e. outcomes by type of surgery, type of complications and case severity level or co-morbidity. Obviously, these are essential data for monitoring surgical outcomes.

Several items relate to manager and physician concerns about the effects of recent changes in the health care system on quality of care and clinical outcomes. The first and most obvious change in Quebec, as in other jurisdictions, has been budget cuts and their possible impact on access and waiting lists. Although not among their top priorities, both groups of respondents are interested in knowing whether outcomes are different according to the length of time between the decision to operate (surgery request) and the actual operation (managers item 16 and physicians items 12 and 24). The second important change in the health care system is called the 'ambulatory shift', that is, a reduction in the use of inpatient care. Again, a number of items relate to that change. For example, the top priority for managers is to be able to distinguish outcomes by type of care (day surgery, short stay, etc.). Both physicians and managers are interested in complications treated on an outpatient basis. Physicians are looking for outcomes according to the length of postoperative stay (item 13), possibly wanting to test whether patients returning home more quickly are worse off.

Some items mentioned by physicians show their particular interest in the process of care. For example, they would like outcomes to be documented according to which day of the week or what time during the day a surgical procedure is performed (items 18 and 19). They also care about the reason for

Table 11.1 Content that managers and physicians want included in surgical outcome measure reports

Priority	Outcomes should be provided …	Score
Managers		
1	By type of care: day surgery, short stay, hospitalization	56
2	Re. complications during the hospitalization	50
3	By type of surgery	47
4	By type of complication	45
5	By case severity level	28
6	By surgical specialty	24
7	By type of anaesthesia	23
8	By degree of emergency at admission	21
9	Re. complications in the 7 days following discharge	17
10	Re. complications treated on outpatient basis	13
11	By age of patient	12
12	By principal diagnosis	12
13	By time spent in the intensive care unit	12
14	By size of hospital	10
15	Re. rehospitalization	8
16	By time since decision to operate	7
Physicians		
1	By type of surgery	62
2	By type of complication	44
3	By age of patient	38
4	By co-morbidity	35
5	By principal diagnosis	33
6	Re. complications needing a treatment	31
7	By degree of emergency at admission	18
8	Re. complications treated on outpatient basis	15
9	By pre-operative hospital stay	14
10	By degree of anaesthetic risk	13
11	Re. complications common to different specialties	12
12	By delay between surgery request and surgery	12
13	By postoperative stay	12
14	By diagnosis-related group	12
15	By hospital university affiliation	12
16	For hospitalization via emergency room	11
17	Re. complications during the hospitalization	10
18	By length of stay	10
19	By time of day of the operation	10
20	By day of the week of the operation	10
21	Re. rehospitalization	9
22	By reason of pre-operative delay	9
23	Comparing with other hospitals	9
24	By delay between diagnosis and treatment	8
25	By specialty	7

pre-operative delay (item 22).

There were fewer items that managers and physicians mentioned regarding the form of presentation of the outcome reports, which was the second theme discussed (Table 11.2). Both groups would like reports to include figures, tables and main results, although these items have a higher priority for physicians than managers. A detailed description of the methodology used for measuring outcomes is also important for both groups of respondents.

Table 11.2 Form of presentation that managers and physicians want surgical outcome measure reports to take

Priority	Reports should ...	Score
Managers		
1	Be concise, yet complete	55
2	Include a detailed description of the methodology	51
3	Provide quantitative data	49
4	Include a description of relations between factors	44
5	Use a combination of different forms of presentation (figures, tables, main results)	38
6	Provide an interpretation of the results	37
7	Provide the identity of hospitals of comparison	31
8	Present questions raised by the results	19
Physicians		
1	Include figures	70
2	Include tables	63
3	Present main results	56
4	Be accompanied by software to do own analysis	49
5	Offer the possibility of obtaining details on demand	42
6	Include a detailed description of the methodology	35

Differences between the two groups also exist. The top priority for managers is to have a concise but complete report. Contrary to physicians, they are very interested in having clues as to the interpretation of the data and the questions raised (items 4, 6 and 8). The physicians, on the other hand, would like to have access to more details than provided in a standard report (item 5) and be able to use software to do their own analysis of the data (item 4).

The characteristics of the information to be included in outcome reports was the third theme discussed with the consulted managers and physicians. There was a large consensus among participants of both groups on the important items, so no votes were needed (hence no table). In descending order of priority, participants felt that the data should be recent and scientifically valid and that confidentiality or anonymity should be protected at different levels (patient, physician, hospital).

On the latter issue, managers said that they did not need to be able to attribute particular outcomes to specific physicians. They felt that if managers could make this connection, it would create serious tensions in their organizations. They preferred to consider the physicians as a group (yet documenting outcomes by specialty) and not be involved in discussions among physicians. However, the anonymity of hospitals is not necessary for managers. On the contrary, they think it would be useful to know which hospitals they are compared to. Although physicians agree with managers about the confidentiality of the data concerning each physician, they think that hospitals should not be identified.

The fourth and final theme examined in the nominal group meetings concerned the priority of types of surgical procedures for which outcomes should be documented (Table 11.3). Few suggestions were made by the participants. The main similarity between the two groups is that the procedures studied should be those that use more resources, either because they are frequent and costly to perform, or because their complications themselves are serious and costly to treat. Another criteria for selecting the surgeries that should be monitored relates to the 'ambulatory shift' mentioned above: either procedures for which hospital stay has been greatly reduced (managers' top priority) or those done as day surgery (physicians' last priority).

Table 11.3 Priority of types of surgical procedures which managers and physicians want outcome measure reports to focus on

Priority	Surgical procedures should be those ...	Score
Managers		
1	For which hospital stay has been greatly reduced	69
2	With a large volume	59
3	Using new techniques	50
4	Whose complications are costly	47
5	Requiring an important use of resources	43
6	Whose complications are preventable	37
Physicians		
1	That are frequent	70
2	Whose complications are costly	63
3	Whose complications are serious	56
4	Using well established techniques	49
5	Done in day surgery	42

An important difference in points of view between the two groups was whether new or old procedures should be prioritized. Managers thought that new techniques should be monitored in priority in order to adjust them quickly. Physicians felt instead that it would be more fair to look at well-established procedures, because measuring outcomes when a new technique is not fully mastered does not reflect the true quality of care that can be attained.

Discussion

To some extent, the results of this study are consistent with suggestions found in the literature about transfer of research into practice (Lomas, 1997) and wishes commonly expressed by decision-makers about outcome information systems (recent, valid data, etc.). But the study goes beyond general considerations by providing a good understanding of the similarities and differences between manager and physician preferences. In that sense, our study may contribute to the development of clinical indicators that are relevant to decision-makers and that are presented in a way that ensures their effective use.

Essentially, managers and physicians want clear and detailed information that allows them, from their own perspectives, to make the appropriate decisions regarding the type of care to be provided to particular groups of patients. Although the focus of this study was on surgical outcomes, many of our findings are relevant to other types of care.

A particular concern of managers and physicians that largely transcends the field of surgery is monitoring quality of care and patient outcomes following changes in the health care system. This has drawn considerable attention in recent years (Mitchell et al., 1997; Aiken et al., 1997). The most obvious changes are budget cuts and reduction in personnel, 'ambulatory shift', decrease in hospital length of stay and decentralization of services to other settings than inpatient care. An important challenge will be to adapt existing information systems or design new ones that can fulfil decision-makers' needs in this new environment. For example, hospital-based information systems are becoming insufficient in a context where treatments are either initiated, completed or even fully provided outside the hospital. Efficient links between health care delivery settings, including outpatient clinics and even patients' homes, will have to be developed if managers and physicians want a comprehensive picture of the outcomes of the care for which they are responsible. While changes in health care systems are rapidly occurring in many countries, it does not seem that outcome information systems are following at the same pace. Investments will have to be made in this area to adapt to the new information needs created by budget cuts and health system restructuring.

Manager and physician preferences about outcome reports that were gathered here are not necessarily complete: they are those that were expressed spontaneously by the persons consulted. Participants were not asked to express their opinion on the importance of postsurgical complications in evaluating hospital performance. It is possible that other items not mentioned during the group meetings may also be of interest to potential users of outcome reports. In this sense, the next steps in our study, where hospital-specific reports will actually be sent to managers and physicians for their comments and then adjusted accordingly, will be a useful complement to understanding the information needs of decision-makers.

Finally, the consultations we conducted confirmed that managers and physicians have similar but distinctive information needs. If we are to succeed in developing performance information reports and systems that are useful to decision-makers, these differences will have to be taken into account.

References

Aiken, L.H., Sochalski, J. and Lake, E.T. (1997), 'Studying Outcomes of Organizational Change in Health Services', *Medical Care*, 35, 11, Supplement, NS6–NS18.

Billi, J.E., Durand-Arenas, L., Wise, C.G. et al. (1992), 'The Effects of a Low-Cost Intervention Program on Hospital Costs', *Journal of General Internal Medicine*, 7 (4), pp.411–17.

Delbeck, A.L. and Van de Ven, A.H. (1971), 'A Group Process Model for Problem Identification and Program Planning', *Journal of Applied Behavioral Science*, 7, pp. 466–92.

Dyck, F.J., Murphy, F.A., Murphy, J.K. et al. (1977), 'Effect of Surveillance on the Number of Hysterectomies in the Province of Saskatchewan', *The New England Journal of Medicine*, 296 (23), pp. 1326–8.

Flood, A.B., Shortell, S.M. and Scott, W.R. (1994), 'Organizational performance: managing for efficiency and effectiveness' in S.M. Shortell and A.D. Kaluzny (eds), *Health Care Management: Organization Design and Behavior*, 3rd edn, Delmar, Albany, New York.

Grady, M.L., Bernstein, J. and Robinson, S. (1993), *Putting Research to Work in Quality Improvement and Quality Assurance*, Agency for Health Care Policy and Research, US Government of Health and Human Services, Washington, DC.

Klein, R. (1996), 'The NHS and the New Scientism: Solution or Delusion?', *QJM*, 89 (1), pp. 85–7.

Kroenke, K. and Pinholt, E.M. (1990), 'Reducing Polypharmacy in the Elderly: a Controlled Trial of Physician Feedback', *Journal of the American Geriatric Society*, 38 (1), pp. 31–6.

Leggat, S.G., Narine, L., Lemieux-Charles, L. et al. (1998), 'A Review of Organizational Performance Assessment in Health Care', *Health Services Management Research*, 11, pp. 3–23.

Lomas, J. (1997), *Pour améliorer la diffusion et l'utilisation des résultats de la recherche dans le secteur de la santé: la fin des dialogues de sourds*, Centre of Health Economics and Policy Analysis, McMaster University, Hamilton, Ontario.

Manheim, L.M., Feinglass, J., Hugues, R. et al. (1990), 'Training House Officers to Be Cost Conscious: Effects of an Educational Intervention on Charges and Length of Stay', *Medical Care*, 28 (1), pp. 29–42.

Maynard, A. (1997), 'Evidence-based Medicine: an Incomplete Method for Informing Treatment Choices', *Lancet*, 349, 9045, pp. 126–8.

Mitchell, P.H., Heinrich, J., Moritz, P. and Hinshaw, S. (1997), 'Outcome Measures and Care Delivery Systems – Introduction and Purposes of Conference', *Medical Care*, 35, 11, Supplement, NS1–NS5.

Rainwater, J.A., Romano, D. and Antonius, D.M. (1998), 'The California Hospital Outcomes Project: How useful is California's report card for quality improvement?', *Journal on Quality Improvement*, 24 (1), pp. 31–9.

Sicotte, C., Champagne, F., Contandriopoulos, A.P. et al. (1998), 'A Conceptual Framework for the Analysis of Health Care Organizations' performance', *Health Services Management Research*, 11, pp. 24–41.

Wennberg, J.E., Blowers, L., Parker, R. and Gittelsohn, A.M. (1997), 'Changes in Tonsillectomy Rates Associated with Feedback and Review', *Pediatrics*, 59 (6), pp. 821–6.

12 Performance Indicators: A Patient-centred Approach

ANNE LUDBROOK AND COLIN GORDON
Health Economics Research Unit, University of Aberdeen

Introduction

The history of the use of performance indicators in the NHS reveals that they have suffered from many of the recognized defects of such systems. Indeed, the current proposals for a revised framework continue to reflect some of these problems (NHS Executive 1998). This issue would be less important if the nature of the performance targets did not affect management behaviour. A recent survey of a sample of NHS hospital managers, reported here, shows that target setting does influence behaviour and it follows that the wrong targets may detract from rather than promote the pursuit of efficiency (or other objectives).

One of the most serious failures of the performance review system is the lack of integration between the different performance indicators which are necessary in an organization with multiple objectives and multiple outputs. It has been argued that this is too difficult to achieve, but the potential for divergent performance on different indicators is clear (Ferguson and McGuire, 1984; Clatworthy and Mellett, 1997). In this paper, it is argued that developments in clinical guidelines and standard setting offer a basis for a more patient-centred approach and that costs and outcomes could more easily be integrated at this level.

This chapter is concerned with efficiency, although it is recognized that other objectives, such as equity, may also be pursued. The focus is upon systems of performance review in secondary care and the extent to which they are designed to improve the effectiveness and efficiency of the health service in terms of the health outcome for patients. The first section sets out the problem from the perspective of economics. It identifies the features of the health care

Managing Quality: Strategic Issues in Health Care Management, H.T.O. Davies, M. Tavakoli, M. Malek, A.R. Neilson (eds), Ashgate Publishing Ltd, 1999.

sector that give rise to the need for performance indicators and incentives to promote efficiency. This is followed by a brief and critical review of the use of performance indicators within the NHS. The third section reports some relevant findings from a survey of Scottish hospital managers. The final section considers proposals for developing a new approach to performance indicators.

The Nature of the Problem

One of the fundamental tenets of economics is that resources are scarce. Using resources in one particular way implies that they are not available for an alternative use and the benefit that the alternative use would have provided is lost. This forgone benefit is the economists' notion of opportunity cost. If society is to maximize the benefit achieved from available resources then the benefit derived from any particular use must exceed the opportunity cost (allocative efficiency) and the resources employed to achieve the benefit must be minimized (technical efficiency).

In the private sector, competitive markets for both product outputs and shareholder funding are assumed to result, at least where significant market imperfections do not exist, in resources being utilized in both an allocatively and technically efficient manner. Although the conditions for a perfectly competitive market rarely obtain, nevertheless, private markets do work despite considerable imperfections.

Consumers (and potential consumers) can directly observe the merits of a private company's product and compare it with competing products. They can then make an informed consumption choice based on this comparison and if they are dissatisfied with the company's performance as regards either product type, quality or price they possess the ultimate sanction of taking their custom elsewhere. As a result, company managers monitor the market in order to ensure that they are producing the right products and selling them at prices the consumers are willing to pay. Hence, competitive output markets help to ensure that resource allocation reflects consumer preferences and that production is technically efficient.

The competitive market for funds means that shareholders (and potential shareholders) demand information from the company managers which details the use the managers have made of their funds as well as the resulting return or profit earned. The shareholders use this information in order to assess the performance of the management in utilizing their funds and if they are unhappy with their performance in this respect they withdraw their funds by selling their shareholding. Within the private sector, internal reporting systems have been developed which allow managers to quantify, and where possible control for, the factors which contribute to the overall level of profit earned. These factors include turnover, direct costs and indirect costs and targets can be set for their overall levels as well as for their constituent elements. To the extent that the profits earned by private sector firms are indicators of both allocative and technical efficiency, the competitive market for shareholders' funds helps to ensure that resources are allocated and used efficiently.

The health care sector is characterized by market imperfections to the extent that it is not possible to have anything close to a perfectly competitive market. The intrinsic characteristics of health care that lead to market failure have been defined as uncertainty of illness incidence, external effects in consumption and asymmetry of information (Evans, 1984). Other imperfections may be observed in particular health care systems, but these can be traced to institutional responses to the problems arising from these three features.

Recent reforms of the NHS, with the creation of the internal market, were an attempt to introduce a form of managed competition into the NHS, in the belief that this would produce efficiency gains. However, the extent of any competition in such a system is also limited by the nature of the product. In particular, the fact that location and timing are important factors in the consumption of health care limits the extent to which substitution between providers can take place. As a result, competitive output markets generally do not and cannot exist in the health sector, with providers operating as effective local monopolies. Taxpayers could, in theory, withdraw funding from the health service through the political process but this is a very remote sanction. Current proposals to improve the NHS are 'based on co-operation, not competition' (Scottish Office, 1997).

In the absence of competitive markets there is an obvious need for performance measures or indicators which allow the various interest groups, such as potential users, users and taxpayers, to assess the efficiency with which health service managers are utilizing resources. In theory, at least, making interest groups more informed regarding the performance of health service managers should result in resources being used in an efficient manner. As is the case in the private sector, the design of external reporting systems has a profound impact on internal control mechanisms as managers become sensitive to the external indicators to which they are held to account.

Performance indicators are needed at different levels, for different purposes and to satisfy the needs of different interest groups. This has led to the development of a wide range of performance indicators, which are reviewed briefly in the next section. It is argued that insufficient attention has been paid to ensuring that performance indicators meet the purposes for which they are required; in particular, the promotion of efficiency.

The NHS Response – A Brief Review of Performance Indicators

From the perspective of economics, the principal objective of the UK NHS is to utilize the resources at its disposal in both an allocatively and technically efficient manner. Failure to use resources efficiently is not only wasteful in financial terms but has implications for patient care through reductions in the quantity and quality of care provided. Given this objective, and in light of the absence of competitive market pressure as outlined above, it is essential to devise robust and accurate efficiency measures, or performance indicators, which can promote the development of efficiency within the NHS.

Attempts to devise systems of performance indicators, for the NHS and for other public services, have been characterized by a number of problems (Smith, 1993). From the perspective adopted for this paper, the first concern is that the NHS has multiple objectives and multiple outputs. Performance indicators need to fulfil several purposes and no means has been developed to integrate the whole system; that is, to identify how much performance loss on one indicator would be traded for improvement on another, in order to produce an overall assessment of performance across a range of indicators. Little attention has been given to the potential conflicts between objectives.

Secondly, and to the extent that performance indicators are concerned with efficiency, the definition of efficiency is poor and is often restricted purely to cost. This relates to the previous point in that efficiency requires costs and outcomes to be considered together. Different users require different kinds of efficiency information. Commissioners of services need information on costs and health outcomes across a range of services in order to allocate resources between them efficiently. At the operational level, managers require information that will enable them to improve the technically efficiency with which units of output are produced. Their data requirements are quite different and are often unrecognized.

Thirdly, there are a number of problems related to measurement. Proxies are used because suitable measures are not available; not only do these not measure what they purport to measure but frequently movements in the performance indicator can be ambiguous. Measurement of particular aspects of performance can introduce bias as other aspects of performance are ignored.

The first comprehensive package of performance indicators was published in 1983 (Department of Health and Social Services, 1983). Although it was stated that the indicators needed to be considered as a package, the range and complexity of indicators led managers to focus on the published rankings. By 1988, over 2,500 individual indicators were published. This tended to suggest that, rather than a clearly focused attempt at performance measurement, a scatter gun approach had been taken (Ham and Woolley, 1996). Although efforts were made to present the information in a user-friendly fashion and to provide advice on their analysis, it was not easy for the users to identify those indicators which highlight good or bad relative performance.

The rationale behind the indicators package published in 1983 was that it would augment the existing systems of financial control and accountability. The indicators were to be seen as a starting point in assessing performance. However, it is difficult to see how these indicators could be used to promote more efficient use of resources. The majority of the indicators were based on either clinical activity within hospital specialties, for example average length of stay and annual throughput per bed, or focused on hospital financial performance such as cost per case and cost per inpatient day. Any differences in performance would be impossible to interpret without detailed case mix data.

The introduction of the NHS Efficiency Index could be seen as an attempt to produce an overall assessment of performance. At the same time, a shift was taking place away from performance indicators primarily for the use of managers and towards greater public accountability. The NHS produced other performance tables, relating particularly to guarantees in the Patient's Charter. The NHS Chief Executive has been quoted as stating that it would be too complicated to correlate performance on financial targets and NHS league tables (cited in Clatworthy and Mellett, 1997). However, the objectives underlying Patient's Charter guarantees may conflict with other aspects of performance. A good example of this is the use of waiting time targets. Here the objective is clear and readily monitored but has little to do with efficiency as the target waiting times take no account of the benefit to patients. This can result in patients with low clinical priority taking precedence over more urgent cases because of the waiting time target.

The index is open to a number of criticisms (Appleby 1997a and 1997b) and its use is to be abandoned. The method by which the index is constructed gives an incentive for providers to concentrate on those activities which are both included in the index and which are heavily weighted. The index is not sophisticated enough to cover all the types of activity undertaken within the

NHS. Hence, innovative health care provision at the hospital level which adds to overall efficiency but which is not considered in the construction of the index will not be recognized. It is also the case that the included activity types are not given equal weighting. This is a particular problem if the omitted or lowly weighted types of activity are more efficient than those that are highly weighted.

Importantly, the index takes no account of changes in case mix over time. Changes in a purchaser or provider index score may be due to changes in demographic or epidemiological factors rather than due to planned action on their part. The index deals poorly with the substitutability between some types of activity. For example, it may make sense on efficiency grounds to substitute day case work for inpatient stays for certain conditions. However, if both types of treatment are given equal weights in the index managers have no incentive to make this change.

One of the serious omissions in the systems of performance indicators was the lack of information on outcomes. Some moves have been made towards rectifying this situation, particularly in Scotland. Since 1992, the Clinical Resource and Audit Group (CRAG) have promoted work on outcome indicators. The fifth report, produced in 1996, included emergency readmission rates after surgery for selected procedures, activity data for selected procedures and cancer survival rates (CRAG, 1996). Similar types of indicators are included in the current proposals for performance assessment. However, the CRAG report comes with a strong caveat:

> no conclusions should be drawn from any of the comparisons in this report about the quality or the efficacy of the treatment provided ... There may well be important differences ... but these cannot be identified from these comparatively crude comparisons (op. cit., p. 3).

The current proposals in the Green Paper (NHS Executive, 1998) have sets of indicators relating to six areas; health improvement, fair access, effective delivery of appropriate health care, efficiency, patient and carer experience, and health outcomes of NHS care. This is described as a framework for performance assessment and the discussion of the proposals recognizes, for example, that the pursuit of quality and efficiency must go together. There is no mechanism to relate together different aspects of performance, however.

Some of the proposals for efficiency indicators represent an improvement over past systems, but more generally there is a failure to recognize that efficiency encompasses both inputs and outputs. The example given for an efficiency indicator under care of the elderly is the rate of discharge home within 56 days of admission with fractured neck of femur. A high rate may be a desirable objective but it cannot be said to be efficient unless there is also information about the cost of achieving it and about adverse effects, such as readmission to NHS or other care settings. The proposed high level indicators are recognized as being limited by information readily available and a more outcomes focused approach is promised as data become available. However, outcomes indicators appear to be seen as a separate category within the framework and there is no discussion of how these could be linked with other indicators.

The literature on performance indicators in both public and private sectors clearly sets out the difficulties inherent in ensuring that they do promote the desired objectives. The next section discusses some results of a survey of hospital managers relating to their responses to performance indicators and their views on how efficiency could be promoted.

Bed Management Survey

Recently, a study was conducted by the authors on behalf of the Scottish Office Management Executive which examined hospital bed management in Scottish NHS hospitals and which included interviews with managers with responsibilities at both strategic and operational levels at 12 hospitals. The interviews covered a range of topics concerning efficient bed management. Those which are particularly relevant to this discussion are the use of external and internal target setting and the development of clinical guidelines.

The study was commissioned with particular emphasis placed on occupancy and length of stay as indicators of relative efficiency. It became clear that, although these traditional performance indicators might be raised if a hospital was considered to have a real problem, they were rarely part of routine target setting. As far as external target setting was concerned, the main purchasers (Health Boards) tended to focus on activity levels, waiting time guarantees and financial targets.

Hospital managers respond to externally set targets by setting internal targets in order to facilitate their attainment. Therefore, internal performance review would be driven by activity levels, waiting times and financial targets. These would be seen as linked because failure to meet activity or waiting time targets could attract financial penalties. Although most managers said that they would do some kind of comparison of their performance with Scottish averages on indicators such as occupancy or length of stay, it appeared that changes in working practice were more likely to occur where this was necessary to ensure that activity levels were achieved. This could mean that specialties that were behind on contract performance would have their resources protected irrespective of whether their performance was due to inefficiency. The potential for perverse incentives could be great.

Most managers were sceptical about the quality of the routine data available for making comparisons, citing problems such as the way in which costs are apportioned varying across different hospitals and variations in organization that can distort the statistics. Occupancy statistics were criticized on the basis that they are distorted by bed borrowing between specialties and that they are based on a bed count at midnight. The concentration on percentage occupancy may be misleading as high occupancy is more difficult to achieve with a smaller bed complement. The number of beds empty may be more relevant. Bed borrowing also distorts cost data as the ward costs incurred by boarded out patients will appear in the budgets of the host specialties but the activity data will not. The level of detail routinely available can also reduce the relevance of data:

> it is very difficult to compare because of the way that adult medicine is organized. All the patients are triaged into specialties, although they are still called general medicine.

The performance review system and the poor quality of the indicators may encourage managers to spend as much effort on explaining away variations in performance as on attempting to improve performance. In the words of one manager: 'we have a unique set of circumstances but then every Trust would say that, wouldn't they?'. Time and effort is directed at seeking explanations for variances rather that improving efficiency.

One of the managers with strategic responsibilities argued that purchasers should have been setting standards by procedure with respect to factors such as outcomes and length of stay. This was one of the few hospitals where attempts were being made internally to work with clinicians to develop condition specific comparisons. In other places, managers at the operational level were aware that efficiency improvements could be obtained by moving in this direction but were unable to implement the necessary changes. For example, a nurse manager said:

> With pre-assessment, whilst we can prepare to discharge hopefully the patient earlier, we still then have to overcome old traditions of consultants who want to

give their patients 14 days regardless of what services have been put in place to accommodate them back home.

A directorate manager, asked about guidelines for length of stay, commented:

> that is something that the clinicians need to look at in more detail because we could have three different clinicians doing the same procedure and they would all stay for different lengths of stay but I think that that is something that the clinical director could perhaps tackle with his colleagues. I think they take that more kindly from another white coat than they do from a manager.

Given that managers do respond to externally set targets, it is important that targets based on performance indicators do not give managers incentives to undertake behavior which is counter to the attainment of efficiency. Ideally, performance indicators should also provide a basis upon which efficiency can be improved. Performance indicators based purely on hospital or specialty activity and finance are unlikely to promote the attainment of efficiency. In order to be effective in driving the development of the NHS towards increasing efficiency, indicators must provide a guide as to the action to be taken by hospital managers to improve efficiency. Current indicators can highlight specific problems but, without further detailed investigation, provide no guidance as to the required response.

Two of the hospitals in the sample were involved in a research project developing critical care pathways. In the final section of this chapter, these are considered as a way forward in performance assessment.

The Way Forward?

From the preceding sections it can be seen that past approaches to performance indicators in the NHS have suffered from a number of problems: in particular, failure to define efficiency adequately; failure to integrate issues of cost, activity and outcomes; and failure to give managers useful information on how efficiency could be improved. These problems appear to be carried forward in current proposals.

In this final section of the chapter, our main concern is to deal with how efficiency could be promoted by a new approach to performance measurement that would integrate cost and outcome data. One possibility would be a more sophisticated analysis of the existing indicators by the use of techniques such as Data Envelopment Analysis (DEA) (Townsend and Harris, 1997). Whilst this provides a theoretical framework for analysing inputs and outputs, in practice the quality of the underlying data means that many of the problems with traditional performance indicators would remain. It is also the case that DEA assesses relative efficiency. The nature of the analysis is such that outliers may be identified as efficient simply because they have no comparators. As with other performance indicators, the results of DEA will identify potential problems but will not provide guidance to managers on the action required. This would require further investigation.

The critical problem with the performance indicators used since the 1980s has been that they focus on aggregate activity at the hospital or specialty level. The overall objective of improving efficiency was never translated into specific terms that were relevant to each area of activity. Technical efficiency within a hospital setting requires that each individual case should be treated efficiently and the performance of hospitals should be judged on the extent to which this is achieved.

This is by no means a new idea. The same point was made in the context of the reforms that introduced the internal market:

> the ultimate aim of information is to improve the effectiveness of the health services in terms of the health outcome for patients. This suggests that information should assist doctors, nurses and other professionals in delivering the most efficient service to patients, within resource constraints, and subject to whatever criteria of equity are deemed appropriate (Smith 1990).

What has happened since then is that considerable effort has been devoted to improving the effective delivery of health care, through the development of clinical standards, guidelines and clinical audit and the promotion of evidence based medicine. This has proceeded in a rather piecemeal fashion. The Green Paper points out that the lack of appropriate indicators for the effective delivery of care highlights a lack of national monitoring of clinical standards. Furthermore, although information for purchasers is promoting considerations of cost-effectiveness, relatively little attention has been paid to routinely linking the development of standards and guidelines with cost information.

Whilst the greater emphasis being placed on outcome indicators is to be welcomed, if these are restricted to broad comparisons across providers then they will still be inadequate as a basis upon which managers can act to improve efficiency. As the authors of the CRAG report indicated, there are too many possible reasons for variations. As reported in the previous section, some managers identified the need for condition specific comparisons to provide a basis for improving efficiency. This would certainly reduce the scope for explaining away differences in performance. However, it may be possible to go further than this and compare local practice with national standards or guidelines.

In the USA, managed care has been developed with the aim of limiting costs without compromising quality of care. It appears to have had some success, but the evidence depends upon the institutional setting, which is clearly different from the UK (Robinson and Steiner, 1997). The approach makes extensive use of guidelines and protocols and it is this feature that may be most useful to examine in a UK context. Two of the sample hospitals reported on earlier, were involved in a research study relating to the use of integrated care pathways, or critical care pathways. These have been proposed as a way of encouraging the use of guidelines (Campbell et al., 1998). They have been defined as structured multidisciplinary care plans detailing the essential steps in the care of patients with a specific clinical problem.

Performance indicators focused initially at the level of individual patient care should be more effective in promoting technical efficiency. Such indicators could be based upon the establishment of critical care pathways which would reflect evidence based definitions of good clinical practice. As these currently stand, they would promote more effective delivery of health care; in order to promote efficiency, the standard setting or guidelines process must take account of resource use.

The integration of costs or resource use into the critical care pathways would need to happen at two levels. The development of the original standards or guidelines should be based routinely on considerations of cost-effectiveness and not just effectiveness. The care plans developed on the basis of such guidelines could be costed in order to produce an expected cost per case. It should be noted that the expected cost should have nothing to do with comparative efficiency but should represent a standard to be attained, although attaining this will depend upon having agreed costs for the resource inputs identified.

It is recognized that not all patients fit neatly into a set of guidelines. Just as the clinical care of patients will sometimes vary for good reason, so will the costs of treating them. The hospital performance indicators based on such an approach could take this into account by setting targets in terms of the percentage of patients treated within guidelines and an associated deviation from expected unit cost. One of the advantages of the approach would be that the care plans themselves would provide a basis for examining such variations. Critical care pathways are intended to facilitate the audit of clinical practice and they are intended to have a prospective role.

This approach to developing performance indicators would have the advantage of providing a direct link with clinical activity at the individual patient level and would be based on standards reflecting good practice against which the process of care could be audited. Such an approach would facilitate the integration of different information systems and would work with existing trends towards evidence based practice, the development of guidelines and clinical audit.

The difficulties that face managers in making use of information on clinical effectiveness have been highlighted recently (Walshe and Ham, 1997). A recent survey of acute hospitals found that 19 per cent of hospitals had a written strategy for developing clinical guidelines and a further 45 per cent were developing them (Renvoize et al., 1998). This suggests that the framework for using clinical effectiveness information is being put in place at hospital level, although the evidence base used in the development of guidelines was variable.

Although the proposals in the Green Paper (NHS Executive, 1998) are subject to some of the same criticisms as previous systems of performance assessment (McKee and Sheldon, 1998; Appleby, 1998), they also include some indicators that are more relevant at the operational level but not in systematic way. Examples of indicators that would more clearly direct managers to areas requiring attention include the rate of discharge within a specified time, day case rates, use of inappropriate surgical techniques and emergency readmission rates. Such indicators cannot inform managers whether the area of concern is inefficient or under resourced, however.

The intention of the proposed framework is that it will highlight gaps in the available information and act as a catalyst for the development work needed to fill these gaps and improve information. This makes it all the more important that the framework should be clear about what indicators are needed rather than what is available. Building upon patient-centred information, as proposed here, appears to fit with the overall aims of the Green Paper framework.

The costs of developing performance indicators have to be taken into account. There is a clear trade off between the complexity of the system and costs. Although the patient-centred approach may appear to require a lot of data, these are already being developed, as evidenced by the growing use of guidelines cited above, and are being evaluated in terms of their benefit to patients. What is proposed is the extension of this work to include cost information. If successful, this approach would also provide answers to the question of *why* practice deviates from the set standard and reduce the costs of investigating such exceptions. The audit focus would ensure that attempts to identify areas to improve performance would be built in.

Patient-centred performance indicators have the potential to meet the criticisms of traditional systems of performance review. Standards of efficiency would be developed at the individual patient level, costs and outcomes would be integrated and commissioning authorities could readily monitor activity levels. The information generated would give a basis for improving efficiency. Whether this potential can be realized, and at a reasonable cost, remains to be established by means of piloting and evaluating the approach.[1]

Note

1 The authors acknowledge funding from the Scottish Office Department of Health, Chief Scientist Office. The views expressed are those of the authors and not the funding body.

Bibliography

Appleby, J. (1997a), *A Measure of Effectiveness?: A critical review of the NHS Efficiency Index*, National Association of Health Authorities and Trusts, Birmingham.

Appleby, J. (1997b), 'Measuring Efficiency in the NHS', *British Journal of Health Care Management*, 3 (2), pp. 75–7.

Appleby, J. (1998), 'Performance Framework', *Health Service Journal*, 5 February, pp. 34–5.

Campbell, H. et al. (1998), 'Integrated Care Pathways', *British Medical Journal*, 316, pp. 133–7.

Clatworthy, M. and Mellett, H. (1997), 'Managing Health and Finance: Conflict or Congruence?', *Public Money and Management*, Oct.–Dec., pp. 41–6.

Clinical Resource and Audit Group (1996), *Clinical Outcomes Indicators*, The Scottish Office, Edinburgh.

Department of Health and Social Services (1983), *Performance Indicators: National summary for 1981*, DHSS, London.

Evans, R.G. (1984), *Strained Mercy. The economics of Canadian health care*, Butterworths, Toronto.

Ferguson, B. and McGuire, A. (1984), *A Short History and Review of the Performance Indicators Issued by the DHSS*, HERU Discussion Paper 9/84, University of Aberdeen.

Ham, C. and Woolley, M. (1996), *How Does the NHS Measure up?: Assessing the performance of health authorities*, National Association of Health Authorities and Trusts, Birmingham.

McKee, M. and Sheldon, T. (1998), 'Measuring Performance in the NHS', *British Medical Journal*, 316, p. 322.

NHS Executive (1998), *The New NHS: Modern and Dependable. A national framework for assessing performance*, NHSE, Leeds.

Posnett, J. and Street, A. (1996), 'Programme Budgeting and Marginal Analysis: An Approach to Priority Setting in Need of Refinement', *Journal of Health Services Research and Policy*, 1 (3), pp. 147–53.

Renvoize, E. B. et al. (1998), 'What Are Hospitals Doing About Clinical Guidelines ?', *Quality in Health Care*, 6, pp. 187–91.

Robinson, R. and Steiner, A. (1997), 'Managed Care. Just Ask US', *Health Service Journal*, 11 December, pp. 24–5.

Scottish Office (1997), *Designed to Care. Renewing the National Health Service in Scotland*, The Stationery Office, Edinburgh.

Smith, P. (1990), 'Information Systems and the White Paper Proposals' in A.J. Culyer, A.K. Maynard and J.W. Posnett (eds), *Competition in Health Care. Reforming the NHS*, Macmillan, London.

Smith, P. (1993), 'Outcome-related Performance Indicators and Organizational Control in the Public Sector', *British Journal of Management*, 4, pp. 135–51.

Townsend, K. and Harris, R. A. (1997), 'Efficiency Rating Factors for Hospitals', *British Journal of Health Care Management*, 3 (5), pp. 254–9.

Walshe, K. and Ham, C. (1997), *Acting on the evidence. Progress in the NHS*, The NHS Confederation, Birmingham.

13 Is Indicator Use for Quality Improvement and Performance Measurement Compatible?

JOANNE LALLY[1] AND RICHARD THOMSON[2]

1   Department of Epidemiology and Public Health, School of Health Sciences,
     The Medical School, University of Newcastle
2   UK QIP

Introduction

Our work in the application of a particular quality indicator programme, the UK QIP (Thomson, McElroy and Kazandjian, 1997) has led us to consider and review the field of indicator use. This chapter draws upon our experience and upon the present literature, although this is an area where a strong evidence base is lacking. We will not cover the issue of indicator development, which includes critically important elements such as the validity and reliability of indicators. This is well addressed elsewhere (Joint Commission on Accreditation of Health Care Organisations, 1990). This chapter will discuss the value of indicators in terms of their capacity to influence the quality of care, drawing upon an historical discussion of the use of indicators in the UK and to a lesser extent in the USA. This approach is taken with the assumption that the ultimate goal of indicator use is to improve the delivery and outcomes of health services, resulting in improved patient care and population health whether, for example, indicators are used as internal tools for quality improvement activity or as external measures to aid choice. The pathway by which different uses of indicators are presumed to lead to quality improvement are however very different, and recognition of this may enable us to identify

Managing Quality: Strategic Issues in Health Care Management, H.T.O. Davies, M. Tavakoli, M. Malek, A.R. Neilson (eds), Ashgate Publishing Ltd, 1999.

the advantages and disadvantages of indicator uses centred around their (potential) impact upon this ultimate goal. This eventually leads to a discussion as to whether different uses of indicators, even if they have the same ultimate goal, are mutually compatible.

What is an Indicator?

The Oxford English Dictionary describes an indicator as 'one who or that which points out, or directs attention, to something', i.e. not as an absolute measure (*The Shorter Oxford English Dictionary*, 1986). The Joint Commission for Accreditation of Health Care Organisations (JCAHO) in the USA defines an indicator as 'a quantitative measure that can be used to monitor and evaluate the quality of important governance, management, clinical and support functions that affect patient outcomes' (Joint Commission on Accreditation of Health Care Organisations, 1990). Those of us concerned with quality improvement in health care are fundamentally interested in change: the quality assurance cycle is a 'change cycle' (Fowkes, 1982). Interestingly, this is one element that the JCAHO definition misses. Monitoring and evaluation may be necessary prerequisites for improvement, but if indicators used in monitoring and evaluation fail to lead to such improvement, or produce unintended change, their value as a quality tool should be questioned.

It is important to recognize that indicators, when used in any field, are rarely if ever a direct measure of quality. Their main strength lies in acting as a flag or screen to identify areas where further investigation or quality assurance activity might be fruitful. Thus, whether use of an indicator leads to quality improvement or not will depend not only on factors inherent to the specific indicator itself, such as whether it is valid and reliable, or whether it is relevant to an area of patient care (or governance) quality, but also on the way in which the indicator is used.

We can consider an indicator or indicator package, such as the Patient's Charter indicators (Department of Health, 1991) or Scottish Clinical Outcome Indicators (Clinical Outcomes Working Group, 1994; Clinical Outcomes Working Group, 1995; Clinical Outcomes Working Group, 1996) as a tool for quality improvement. Any tool in whatever setting can be used appropriately with skill, or can be used poorly with consequent results. Whilst you do not need to be a master craftsman to use a lathe effectively, using it badly can have damaging effects. The same is true of indicators.

Use of Indicators

Whilst the ultimate goal of indicator use may be to improve the quality of care, there are a range of proposed intermediate uses of indicators. Thus indicators can be seen variously as: measures of quality; tools for performance management within the health care system (i.e. measures that enable one sector or group within the NHS to monitor activity of another sector or group and stimulate changes through a system of management and review); measures that can inform and support choices (e.g. that can inform commissioning decisions or patient choice); and as a means of promoting accountability for the proper use of public funds. Put simply, these uses can be divided into *two* fundamentally different tasks, the first in stimulating further investigation and analysis (most clearly consistent with a quality improvement approach), and the second in making judgments, most clearly characterized by the individual choice of a cardiac surgeon by either a patient or referring doctor, based upon a measure of their comparative postoperative mortality rate.

And this is not only an issue that is taxing us within the NHS; there has been a major international explosion of interest in indicator development and use, leading to a bewildering variety of approaches both within and between countries. The USA most clearly illustrates this effect: one commentator has stated that 'the sheer volume of quality monitoring efforts in North America is staggering' (Boyce, 1997). Nonetheless, other countries, Australia in particular, are putting major investment of time and money into the field. In the UK, the latest governmental review and White Paper, *The New NHS: Modern and Dependable* (Department of Health, 1997a) with its plans for quality and clinical governance, and the subsequent *National Framework for Assessing Performance* (Department of Health, 1997b) will further stimulate debate. Furthermore, the recent General Medical Council judgment on the Bristol cardiac surgeons (Treasure, 1998) and the NHS consultation document *A First Class Service: Quality in the New NHS* (Secretary of State for Health, 1998) provided a further drive towards public availability of clinical indicators.

NHS Performance Indicators

The use of performance indicators at a national level within the NHS began in 1983 (Birch and Maynard, 1988; Pollitt, 1985). The original NHS performance indicators were introduced in response to concerns, including those from the Public Accounts Committee, about the absence of any performance measures, leading to a central 'top down' initiative to make better use of routinely collected data to support comparisons at regional and district level. This use of routine NHS data concentrated upon structure and activity measures (including clinical activity, finance, manpower and estate management functions), despite concerns about quality and reliability (Birch and Maynard, 1988). In essence the indicators presented comparative numerical information which allowed health authorities to compare their performance with achievement elsewhere, in areas such as the length of stay of patients, turnover and throughput measures, and cost per case of treating patients.

Initially the data were presented in dense numerical tables, with little evidence of use or interest by clinicians in particular. A major concern was that the data were at least two years old, but the absence of any indicators seen to be of clinical relevance was perhaps of greater importance in explaining the reluctance of clinicians to use the data. Furthermore, there had been little incentive for assuring the quality of the underlying data, leading to inevitable criticism that the figures were unreliable. In 1985 improvements were made in the presentation and timeliness of the indicators, although most of the limitations remained, in particular criticisms of an absence of indicators of effectiveness (Harrison, Hunter, and Pollitt, 1990). The performance indicators were seen to focus principally on efficiency rather than effectiveness and outcomes (Ham, 1992). Despite this, in a survey carried out by CASPE on the usefulness of performance indicators they found that even allowing for the inaccuracies and inconsistencies, the opportunity to make comparisons allowed districts for the first time to begin benchmarking with other districts (Jenkins, Bardsley and Coles, 1987).

In 1986 avoidable deaths indicators (Charlton et al., 1983) were introduced, partly in response to criticisms about absence of effectiveness data, but the problem of small numbers aggregated at a district (resident population) level limited their usefulness. Despite these difficulties the avoidable deaths indicators were seen as potentially very useful, with the advantage over the initial indicators that they are closer to measuring outcomes than the other process orientated performance indicators. At the time, an increase in the amount of data and indicators involved also led to concerns that the volume of data was in itself counter to effective use.

The Patient's Charter

The Griffiths Report in 1983 highlighted the lack of consumer responsiveness of the NHS (Department of Health and Social Security, 1983). With increasing emphasis on accountability of public services, the Patient's Charter, the NHS component of the Citizen's Charter, was introduced in 1991 and included the publication of comparative data for public consumption (Department of Health, 1991). These are now released annually, with hospitals rated on a five point starred scale, leading to the production of ranked data in the media in the form of 'league tables' which ostensibly allow public comparison of several aspects of hospital care including, for example, accident and emergency (A&E) departments.

One of the A&E indicators is the percentage of patients assessed within five minutes of arrival. Whilst the original intent of the indicator was to stimulate more rapid clinical assessment of patients in A&E, there have been a number of problems. At the very least, in order to compare departments appropriately, data must be collected in the same way. However, a national survey of A&E departments has shown that despite the central guidance, data collection varies markedly (Edhouse and Wardrope, 1996). Nor is there a clear definition of 'assessment', the indicator being based on speed rather than quality of assessment. Whilst the concentration upon early assessment may have stimulated wider use of patient triage, whether this has led to *better* patient triage is debatable.

The purpose of triage lies in early assessment in order to classify patients in terms of urgency of need for clinical care, and then treat them according to their need rather than their order of attendance. However triage itself varies, ranging from 'eyeballing', where the nurse greets the patient and rapidly assesses their condition in seconds, to advanced triage which may take up to six minutes and involve a trained nurse performing a detailed history and examination, initiating first aid and making notes with the purpose of classifying the patient according to the urgency of the problem. (Edhouse and Wardrope, 1996). This makes it difficult to compare indicator rates between hospitals as they may reflect very different activities. This is also an example of where use of an indicator that is published, and against which performance is externally judged, can produce perverse incentives. Thus, in some departments there will have been pressure to improve on performance by changing their triage system from advanced triage to 'eyeballing', thus improving the rate but potentially compromising quality of care. Indeed, the survey revealed that some departments were running dual systems, with immediate 'eyeballing' to meet the standard, followed by more comprehensive triage. Of more concern, there appeared to be no correlation between the star rating awarded and the use of full triage or the length of triage (Edhouse and Wardrope, 1996).

The implication of this is that the creation of the pejoratively entitled 'hello nurse' can ensure that the standard is met even if patients receive lower quality assessment and continue to wait prolonged periods for clinical care. This is a clear example of a perverse incentive, due in part to the use of a poorly conceived indicator and in part to its publication for media and public consumption. The publication has indeed led to behaviour change, but not the change that was initially intended. This external inspectoral approach is what Don Berwick (1989) has elegantly described as the 'bad apple' approach, centred around the identification of outliers, leading to unintended consequences.

It is also highly questionable as to how appropriate it is to judge the performance of a complex department by measuring the events that take place in the first five minutes. Whilst this problem has been recognized, and it would appear that this indicator may well be removed from the public performance tables, it nonetheless highlights the problems that can occur as a result of the public availability of measures that will be ranked and used to make judgments. Nonetheless, this foray into comparative data for public consumption has led to calls for similar publication of clinical data, particularly outcomes data, leading to such publication in Scotland (Clinical Outcomes Working Group, 1994; Clinical Outcomes Working Group, 1995; Clinical Outcomes Working Group, 1996) and to a consultation exercise on a similar approach in England and Wales (NHS Executive, 1997). Before considering these, it is pertinent to look at the American experience.

The US Experience

The nature of the highly-fragmented health services in the USA, and the cultural and political milieu within which these exist, and by which they have been shaped, has led to a more consumer-responsive approach within a market-based organization and delivery of health care. Nonetheless, it was the publicly funded sector that created the most dramatic change in terms of publication of indicator data. In 1985, the Health Care Financing Administration (HCFA), the department within the federal government responsible for overseeing the quality and cost-effectiveness of the Medicare and Medicaid programmes, elected (with little consultation or pre-warning) to publish crude mortality rates for hospitals across the USA (US Department of Health and Human Services Health Care Financing Administration, 1987). This decision led both to considerable public interest (Brinkley, 1986) and prominent professional antagonism. Early data were vociferously criticized for the inappropriateness of comparisons based upon crude rates, unadjusted for the case mix variables that could explain much of the observed differences between hospitals (Dubois, 1989).

Thus, the dominant response of health services to the initial publication of this data was that of defensive *explanation* (i.e. those with high rates attempting to explain why they were high, using arguments that they reflected the treatment of older or sicker patients), rather than *exploration* (i.e. attempting to understand the underlying reasons for a particular mortality rate as a means of identifying ways of improving care). Regardless of the intentions of the release of this data, once again this reflects an understandable response to an outlier-based approach (Berwick, 1989).

This stimulated several years' work attempting to develop statistical methods of risk adjustment, with the implicit intention of correcting for patient variables such as age, co-morbidity and severity of illness, in order to allow comparisons that would reflect differences in the quality of antecedent care. Considerable resources were put into this (Iezzoni, 1994). However, in 1993 HCFA suspended its publication of risk-adjusted hospital mortality rates pending review and subsequently decided that the problems were such that they should stop releasing them publicly (Jencks, 1994). Iezzoni has pointed out, from her extensive study of risk adjustment, that to minimize the chance of manipulation the risk-adjusted outcomes data must be perceived as being used in a fair and non-punitive fashion – or at least as providing 'due process' for those contesting any findings (Iezzoni, 1994).

Despite this salutary lesson, the public release of mortality data continues to be suggested and employed as a means of underpinning accountability and choice. Several US states require mortality data to be made publicly available. For example, the state of Pennsylvania has mandated hospitals to provide severity-adjusted data on surgeon specific mortality rates for coronary artery bypass grafting and selected hospital-wide mortality rates in diagnosis related groups (DRG), despite the fact that DRGs were developed to have iso-resource rather than clinical consistency. Annual reports are made available for public consumption (Boyce, 1997).

More recently HCFA has moved into its Health Care Quality Improvement Initiative (HCQII) (Jencks, 1994), away from the 'bad apple' approach to one more concerned with looking at patterns of care and outcomes, and with a more collaborative approach to use of indicator data. The indicators are applied to four major areas – accessibility, appropriateness, outcomes and customer satisfaction. An example of this maturing approach is the 'Co-operative Cardio-vascular Project' which seeks to provide confidential feedback of comparative data to support providers and physicians in improvement work. This approach recognizes the problems experienced with the public release of mortality rates and is predicated upon the view that true and honest self-examination cannot be expected to occur under the threat of publication (Jencks, 1994).

The perceived value of indicators has even penetrated the traditional and long-standing field of accreditation. Long criticized for the nature of the accreditation process, in particular that it provides a snapshot view as to whether an organization can (and not whether it does) deliver high quality care, the Joint Commission on Accreditation of Health Care Organisations began to develop clinical indicators to use within the accreditation process (Joint Commission on Accreditation of Health Care Organisations, 1990; O'Leary, 1987). It has now moved on to accredit indicator packages (including the MHA QIP) in its ORYX initiative (Scrivens 1997). It now requires all of its accredited hospitals to sign up to one of these and, from early 1999, to provide quarterly data which will be monitored by the JCAHO. This could then stimulate 'for cause' accreditation reviews, for example if adverse results or trends are seen. This data will also be publicly disclosed. How this will affect the accreditation process remains to be seen, but it has the potential problems of publicly available data already described.

The Maryland Quality Indicator Project

The public release of hospital mortality data in the mid 1980s had a number of effects. In the State of Maryland, hospitals sought help from the Maryland Hospital Association (MHA) to develop and use indicators that would support them in understanding and improving the quality of their care. This led to the development of the MHA Quality Indicator Project (QIP) (Kazandjian et al., 1993 and 1996; Kazandjian, Wood and Lawthers, 1995). The project developed and piloted a small number of hospital-wide quality indicators, including mortality rates, hospital-acquired infection rates and readmission rates which are collected by participant hospitals quarterly. This data is then forwarded to the MHA, and subsequently fed back to the hospital in a non-threatening way that enables them to be viewed over time and in comparison to other participants. The data have not to date been publicly released and are supported by well developed educational materials. Over 1,100 hospitals are now involved in the project worldwide. The overall aim of this project is to provide hospitals with the information about their rate in comparison to other hospitals in a way that it can be used internally to support ongoing quality programmes. The success of this project is apparent from its wide acceptance and from the extensive case studies demonstrating its capacity to create effective change (Kazandjian et al., 1996; Thomson, McElroy and Kazandjian, 1997). We will return to this, and the UK development of the project, later.

Cardiac Surgery in New York

Since 1989 the New York State Department of Health has collected prospective data on cardiac surgery in New York hospitals (Ciccone and Munshi, 1995). The project is led by a Cardiac Advisory Committee convened by the State Department to advise on information needs and data collection. A detailed risk-adjustment process was developed in order to provide feedback on actual and risk-adjusted cardiac surgery mortality rates. The purpose of the programme was not only to provide feedback of comparative data to hospitals and surgeons, but also to provide public release of data that would help consumers select cardiac surgery centres (Dziuban et al., 1994). Initially information released included volume of cases, crude in-hospital mortality rates and risk-adjusted mortality rates. In 1991 a lawsuit by a newspaper, *Long Island Newsday*, forced the publication of individual surgeons' risk-adjusted data. These are now released for surgeons who have performed at least 200 CABGs in a three year period (Dziuban et al., 1994).

Concern was initially expressed that patients might move away from physicians with a high mortality rate. There was also concern that risk adjustment might not adequately adjust for patients with a higher risk, and that some hospitals or surgeons would avoid high risk patients. In fact no significant movement of patients or referrals away from high rate towards low rate hospitals has been demonstrated and there were remarkable reductions in CABG mortality over the first four years in New York State, most markedly in low volume surgeons (Hannan et al., 1995). However, once again attribution is a problem in such observational data, and there is evidence that rates were falling elsewhere in the US at the same time.

From the beginning of the study low volume surgeons have consistently had higher risk-adjusted mortality rates than high volume surgeons. As a result, some hospitals have restricted the privileges of surgeons, and a number of low volume surgeons ceased operating. Other surgical units reviewed their practices following feedback and made policy or staff changes as a result. For example, St Peter's Hospital, Albany, New York ostensibly had 'high mortality with low risk cases' on risk-adjusted data (Dziuban et al., 1994). Initial clinical response was of scepticism. Further investigation revealed that the major contribution was in fact due to emergency procedures in very high risk patients and appropriate changes in policy led to marked improvements.

Initial press coverage of the public data was more concerned with ranking surgeons, often focusing on differences which were neither clinically nor statistically significant (Chassin, Hannan and DeBuono, 1996). It has subsequently been elegantly shown by Goldstein and Speigelhalter (1996) that the ranking of surgeons using this data is highly problematic. By 1992, after major education of the media on the use and limitations of the indicators, the press accounts began to change from highlighting the ranking of surgeons to describing how hospitals and surgeons used the data to improve the outcomes for their patients (Chassin, Hannan and DeBuono, 1996).

One of the major concerns expressed when looking at the arguments both for and against publication of data such as this, is to what extent their publication may lead to changes that are not in the patients' interest (the concept of perverse incentives) (McKee and Hunter, 1995). For example, would surgeons begin to refuse higher risk patients or patients be rated in a higher risk category before surgery was carried out? Alongside the apparent success of the project, there is some suggestion that data may have been distorted. To the credit of the programme, careful audit of data is undertaken. In the hospitals that have been identified as collecting inaccurate risk data, the risk status of individual patients was enhanced (Chassin, Hannan and DeBuono, 1996). This would have had the effect of reducing the participant's risk-adjusted mortality, as well as distorting the overall model. It is not clear whether this was intentional or not, but the self reports from hospitals involved do indeed suggest that risk status is more frequently recorded as a result of the introduction of the programme, although this may, of course, reflect more accurate recording (Dziuban et al., 1994). However, this potential 'gaming' with data is what would be predicted from the 'bad apple' theory (Berwick, 1989), with public availability and scrutiny of data leading to defensive and self-protective responses. A similar programme within the Department of Veterans Affairs has used paper audits and site visits to high mortality risk-adjusted outliers, raising concerns about a 'bad apple' approach (Daley, 1994).

There is some evidence from the introduction of prospective diagnosis-related group (DRG) payments for Medicare/Medicaid that recording of clinical data may be changed in a way that maximizes income (so called 'DRG creep') (Hsia et al., 1992). It seems highly likely that similar influences will hold sway in outcome indicator projects involving external judgments which have potentially important consequences for hospitals and doctors. It has been suggested in the UK that it may be beneficial for hospitals to have poor comparative figures as this might put pressure on purchasing authorities to increase funding (Bagust, 1996), although it seems much more likely that the converse will be the case with hospitals and clinicians seeking to avoid adverse publicity from 'poor' performance indicators.

Clinical Indicators in the UK

The Health Service in Scotland has produced publicly available comparative clinical outcome indicator reports since 1994, drawing upon the advantages of record linkage within the Scottish morbidity record (an advantage not shared by England and Wales) (Clinical Outcomes Working Group, 1994, 1995 and 1996). Indicators published range from population-based data such as mortality from cervical cancer and incidence of childhood measles, through to hospital-specific indicators such as mortality rates within 30 days of admission for acute myocardial infarction, stroke and fractured neck of femur, D & C rates and emergency readmission rates after surgery. Data presented graphically are standardized for age and sex, and provided with 95 per cent confidence intervals. However, the Chief Medical Officer for Scotland has stated that 'far from assuaging public concern, the publication of outcome indicators may have deepened public anxiety regarding the equity of access to their system' (Chief Medical Officer, 1997).

In England and Wales, a similar approach is under consultation (NHS Executive, 1997). The 15 proposed clinical indicators were said by the Health Minister, Baroness Jay, to mark a move away from judging hospitals solely by management and financial targets, in order to reflect the complexities of health care, such as hospitals working in socially deprived areas with patients who are more at risk in comparison to hospitals who have specialist surgeons performing routine operations (Healy, 1997). It is intended that the chosen indicators will be published annually alongside the Patient's Charter performance data.

One of the major drawbacks will be the completeness and accuracy of the data. The indicators will use routinely collected hospital data from the hospital episodes system, which has notorious inaccuracies. Some information on data quality will be included in the report to allow for identification of areas where the data is incomplete and therefore not wholly appropriate for comparative purposes.

Central Health Outcomes Unit

As well as the clinical indicators package described above, the Central Health Outcomes Unit (CHOU) of the Department of Health in Leeds has been stimulating wider development of outcome indicators that are not restrained by the requirement for routinely available data. Ten multidisciplinary working groups have been created, to identify and appraise candidate indicators and provide guidance on how these might be implemented and developed. The first group to report covered stroke (Working Group on Outcomes Indicators for Stroke, 1997). The stated potential uses of the indicators were for clinical decision making and audit of clinical work, although at present it remains unclear as to how this work will be used.

UK Quality Indicator Project

In this chapter we have discussed one key element of the use of indicators, namely the advantages and disadvantages of using indicators to make judgments, compared to using them as a primary stimulus for quality improvement. The contrast is most apparent from the US experience of the now-abandoned public presentation of hospital wide mortality data by HCFA and the highly successful MHA Quality Indicator Project which relies upon use of anonymized feedback of data to support continuous quality improvement.

As a result of the lessons from the US, the former Northern Regional Health Authority decided to pilot and evaluate the MHA QIP model in British hospitals (Thomson, McElroy and Kazandjian, 1997). This would alleviate the need for *de novo* development of indicators and allow for more rapid assessment of the approach. An evaluation was undertaken which involved two surveys one year apart using semi-structured interviews with a purposive sample of clinicians, managers, project coordinators and purchasers of care; self-completion questionnaires to hospital staff and to those identified as receiving indicator data; a survey of hospital documentary sources; and case studies.

The key findings from this evaluation were:

- the UK QIP was a valued and supported project within the hospitals;
- it takes time to see results from participation – the initial effects are on data quality, changes in clinical practice occur later;
- effective case studies were identified;
- there was a desire for more UK participants to allow for more meaningful UK comparisons;
- there was some desire for extension of the indicators to include some designed specifically for the UK;
- greater support and facilitation within the UK was required.

As a result, funding was obtained from the NHS and the Maryland Hospital Association to set up a UK office and expand the project beyond the pilot sites to the rest of the UK. The UK office, as well as providing participants with the training and support they need to take the project forward within their own organizations, is also encouraging more hospitals to join the project, in order to develop the project further in the light of the results of the evaluation.

Conclusions

The NHS White Paper (Department of Health, 1997a) states that performance in hospitals will be judged by greater use of comparative information and that the new performance framework will encourage greater use of benchmarking. It is hoped that the publication of comparative indicator rates will allow people to compare performance and share best practice.

However, experience elsewhere, and from the UK QIP, suggests that there must be concern about the most effective use of indicator data (Thomson, McElroy and Kazandjian, 1997). Whilst we have concentrated largely on the hospital setting it seems likely that the experience here will be equally applicable to other settings such as primary health care. We believe that the limitations of indicators need to be clearly recognized before they can be used to their fullest effect, in leading to demonstrable change within the context of continuous quality improvement.

The forthcoming use of clinical indicators in England and Wales offers an ideal opportunity to evaluate the different effects of public availability and comparative anonymized feedback. In this era of evidence-based practice, the Department of Health could usefully use this opportunity to set up a randomized controlled trial across England and Wales; unfortunately it is likely that political imperatives will prevent this opportunity from being taken.

Finally, as Jencks (1994) has pointed out using the HCFA experience, the ultimate criterion for the acceptance of a quality indicator is whether it leads to successful quality improvement projects. We would do well to remember this as we make progress with indicator use in the NHS.

References

Bagust, A. (1996), 'League Tables', *British Journal of Hospital Medicine*, 55 (6), pp. 369–70.

Berwick, D.M. (1989), 'Continuous Improvement as an Ideal in Health Care', *New England Journal of Medicine*, 320, pp. 53–6.

Birch, S. and Maynard, A. (1988), 'Performance Indicators' in R. Maxwell (ed.), *Reshaping the National Health Service*, Policy Journals, Oxford.

Boyce, N. (1997), 'North American Insights into Quality and Outcome: Indicators in acute healthcare services' in N. Boyce, J. McNeil, D. Graves and D. Dunt (eds), *Quality and Outcome Indicators for Acute Healthcare Services*, Australian Government, Canberra.

Brinkley, J. (1986), 'US Releasing Lists of Hospitals with Abnormal Mortality Rates', *New York Times*, 12 March.

Charlton, J.R.H., Hartley, R.M., Silver, R. and Holland, W.W. (1983), 'Geographical Variation in Mortality from Conditions Amenable to Medical Intervention in England and Wales', *Lancet*, 1, pp. 691–6.

Chassin, M.R., Hannan, E.I. and DeBuono, B.A. (1996), 'Benefits and Hazards of Reporting Medical Outcomes Publicly', *The New England Journal of Medicine*, 334 (6), pp. 394–8.

Chief Medical Officer (1997), 'From the Chief Medical Officer', *Health Bulletin*, 55 (4), pp. 201–3.

Ciccone, K.R. and Munshi, O.D. (1995), 'Measurable Accountability in an Era of Health Care Reform' in V.A. Kazandjian (ed.), *The Epidemiology of Quality*, Maryland, Aspen.

Clinical Outcomes Working Group (1994), *Clinical Outcome Indicators*, The Scottish Office Clinical Resource and Audit Group, Edinburgh.

Clinical Outcomes Working Group (1995), *Clinical Outcome Indicators*, The Scottish Office Clinical Resource and Audit Group, Edinburgh.

Clinical Outcomes Working Group (1996), *Clinical Outcome Indicators*, The Scottish Office Clinical Resource and Audit Group, Edinburgh.

Daley, J. (1994), 'Criteria by Which to Evaluate Risk-adjusted Outcome Programs in Cardiac Surgery', *Annals of Thoracic Surgery*, 58, pp. 1827–35.

Department of Health (1991), *The Patient's Charter: Raising the standard*, HMSO, London.

Department of Health (1997a), *The New NHS: Modern and Dependable*, Department of Health, London.

Department of Health (1997b), *The New NHS: Modern and Dependable: A National Framework for Assessing Performance*, Department of Health, London.

Department of Health and Social Security (1983), *NHS management inquiry* (Griffiths report), HMSO, London.

Dubois, R. W. (1989), 'Hospital Mortality as an Indicator of Quality' in N. Goldfield and D.B. Nash (eds), *Providing Quality Care: The challenge to clinicians*, American College of Physicians, Philadelphia.

Dziuban, S.W., McIlduff, J.B., Miller, S.J. and Dal Col, R.H. (1994), 'How a New York Cardiac Surgery Program Uses Outcomes Data', *Annals of Thoracic Surgery*, 58, pp. 1871–6.

Edhouse, J.A. and Wardrope, J. (1996), 'Do the National Performance Tables Really Indicate the Performance of Accident and Emergency Departments?', *Journal of Accident and Emergency Medicine*, 13, pp. 123–6.

Fowkes, F.G.R. (1982), 'Medical Audit Cycle', *Medical Education*, 16, pp. 228–38.

Goldstein, H. and Speigelhalter, D.J. (1996), 'League Tables and Their Limitations: Statistical issues in comparisons of institutional performance', *Journal of the Royal Statistical Society A.*, 159 (3), pp. 385–443.

Ham, C. (1992), *Health policy in Britain*, 3rd edn, Macmillan Press Ltd, London.

Hannan, E.L., Siu, A.L., Kumar, D., Kilburn, H. and Chassin, M.R. (1995), 'The Decline in Coronary Artery Bypass Graft Surgery Mortality in New York State', *Journal of American Medical Association*, 273 (3), pp. 209–13.

Harrison, S., Hunter, D.J. and Pollitt, C. (1990), *The Dynamics of British Health Policy*, Routledge, London.

Healy, P. (1997), 'Jay Spells Out Significance of New Indicators', *Health Service Journal*, 17th July, p. 10.

Hsia, D.C., Ahern, C.A., Ritchie, B.P., Moscoe, L.M. and Krushat, W.M. (1992), 'Medicare Reimbursement Accuracy Under the Prospective Payment System 1985 to 1988', *Journal of American Medical Association*, 268 (7), pp. 896–9.

Iezzoni, L.I. (1994), 'Using Risk-adjusted Outcomes to Assess Clinical Practice: An Overview of Issues Pertaining to Risk Adjustment', *Annals of Thoracic Surgery*, 58, pp. 1822–6.

Jencks, S.F. (1994), 'HCFA's Health Care Quality Improvement Program and the Co-operative Cardiovascular Project', *Annals Thoracic Surgery*, 58, pp. 1858–62.

Jenkins, L., Bardsley, M. and Coles, J. (1987), *Use and Validity of NHS Performance Indicators: A national survey*, CASPE Research, London.

Joint Commission on Accreditation of Health Care Organisations (1990), *Primer on indicator development and application*, JCAHO, Chicago.

Kazandjian, V.A., Lawthers, J., Cernak, C.M. and Pipesh, F.C. (1993), 'Relating Outcomes to Processes of Care: The Maryland Hospital Association's Quality Indicator Project (QI Project)', *Joint Commission Journal on Quality Improvement*, 19 (11), pp. 530–8.

Kazandjian, V.A., Thomson, R.G., Law, W.R. and Waldron, K. (1996), 'Do Performance Indicators Make a Difference?', *Joint Commission Journal on Quality Improvement*, 22, pp. 482–91.

Kazandjian, V.A., Wood, P. and Lawthers, J. (1995), 'Balancing Science and Practice in Indicator Development: The Maryland Hospital Association Quality Indicator (QI) Project', *International Journal for Quality in Health Care*, 7, pp. 39–46.

McKee, M. and Hunter, D. (1995), 'Mortality League Tables: Do they inform or mislead?', *Quality in Health Care*, 4, pp. 5–12.

NHS Executive (1997), *Clinical Indicators for the NHS (1994 – 95): A consultation document*, NHS Executive, London.

NHS Executive (1997), *Working Group on Outcomes Indicators for Stroke (1997): Report to the Department of Health*, NHS Executive, London.

O'Leary, D.S. (1987), *The Joint Commission's Agenda for Change*, JCAHO, Chicago.

Pollitt, C. (1985), 'Measuring Performance: A new system for the national health service', *Policy and Politics*, 13, pp. 1–15.

Scrivens, E. (1997), 'Putting Continuous Quality Improvement into Accreditation: Improving approaches to quality assessment', *Quality in Health Care*, 6, pp. 212–8.

Secretary of State for Health (1998), *A First Class Service: Quality in the NHS*, HMSO, London.

The Shorter Oxford English Dictionary (1986), Oxford University Press, Oxford.

Thomson, R.G., McElroy, H. and Kazandjian, V.A. (1997), 'Maryland Hospital Association Quality Indicator Project in the United Kingdom: An approach for promoting continuous quality improvement', *Quality in Health Care*, 6, pp. 49–55.

Treasure, T. (1998), 'Lessons from the Bristol Case', *British Medical Journal*, 316, pp. 1685–6.

US Department of Health and Human Services Health Care Financing Administration (1987), *Medicare Hospital Mortality Information, 1986*, US Government Printing Office, Washington.

14 Published Health Outcomes: Guiding Lights or Wreckers' Lanterns?

HUW T.O. DAVIES,[1] IAIN K. CROMBIE[2] AND
RUSSELL MANNION[3]

1   Department of Management, University of St Andrews
2   Department of Epidemiology and Public Health, University of Dundee,
     Ninewells Hospital and Medical School
3   Centre for Health Economics, University of York

Introduction

Accountability and control of clinical staff are much to the fore in reformed health systems. The rise of managed care in the United States (Robinson and Steiner, 1998) has led to unprecedented attempts at controlling physician behaviour, developments which are being followed closely on this side of the Atlantic. In the United Kingdom, the Labour government (elected in May 1997) have made improving quality a cornerstone of their health strategy. Three major government publications attest to the seriousness of the administration's determination to improve health professionals' performance: the latest White Paper, *The New NHS: Modern and Dependable* (Secretary of State for Health, 1998), the *National Performance Framework* (NHS Executive, 1998) and the consultation paper on quality *A First Class Service* (Secretary of State for Health, 1998).

Numerous different strategies have been proposed to improve clinical performance and strengthen accountability. However, the ready availability of information technology has fuelled a growth in systems which intend to measure and monitor both the quantity and the quality of care. The proliferation of performance indicators, and especially the rising role of health outcomes,

Managing Quality: Strategic Issues in Health Care Management, H.T.O. Davies, M. Tavakoli, M. Malek, A.R. Neilson (eds), Ashgate Publishing Ltd, 1999.

demonstrate a growing concern with external scrutiny in assuring quality and improving performance.

This chapter uses a 'principal-agent' framework to examine some of the underlying problems of physician control and to assess the role of some of the possible solutions to these problems. It is aimed at putting the use of performance indicators when used as instruments of control (including the growing use of health outcomes) into a broader theoretical and practical context.

The Principal-agent Problem

The 'principal-agent framework' is a way of looking at important reciprocal relationships within and between organizations: agents act on behalf of principals to achieve some end. Health care is characterized by many different sorts of principal-agent relationships (Propper, 1995; Smith et al., 1997). Using this framework, for example, doctors (and other health care professionals) are *agents* used to bring about health gains for patients; health service managers (whether in provider units or purchasing authorities) are the *principals* on whose behalf these agents are striving. In turn, health care managers and health authorities can also be seen as the agents of government (another principal). Thus health systems are made up of many, diverse and overlapping principal-agent relationships. The 'principal-agent framework' is a way of examining how and why agents may fail to perform as principals might wish. It is used to shed light on the ways in which principals seek to ensure that agents are controlled and accountable.

Difficulties occur in the principal-agent relationship because of incongruities and asymmetries between them. Were principals and agents identical in their knowledge, beliefs, attitudes and objectives then few problems would arise. It is differences between principals and agents that create the need for control mechanisms and systems of accountability.

Principals and agents may have largely overlapping objectives or widely divergent ones. In many cases it may be hard to tell which because the objectives and motivations of both agents and principals may be implicit and submerged rather than obvious. Once divergence exists between principals and their agents the possibility arises that agents will seek to meet their own objectives in preference to those of the principal. The problem is compounded by an asymmetry of information: agents invariably know much more about their own actions and consequent outcomes than any principal. Thus there exists the potential for opportunism on the part of agents, exploiting the powerful position afforded them by the principal's limited view. For example, the NHS has until comparatively recently been a service-led organization, with doctors exploiting their dominant position to define what they see as appropriate service patterns. Many health service reforms (in Britain and elsewhere) have been aimed at curbing this exploitation of agency power by trying to ensure that services are provided on the basis of community need.

Approaches to Agent Control

Principals face a number of options in seeking to overcome the potential for agent waywardness. Which routes are chosen or, more likely, the balance between several approaches, is an important consideration in planning any strategy for performance enhancement in health care.

The first option open to principals is to foster a greater congruence of goals between themselves and their agents. The greater the overlap in objectives (i.e. the better the agreement of their utility functions) the happier the principal can be that the agent will act faithfully, which then obviates the need for additional control. Of course, ascertaining the extent to which agents' objectives truly do reflect those of the principal may be difficult (if not impossible) to determine.

A second approach to improving agents' performance in line with principals' objectives is the development of a market whereby agents compete for the attention of principals. Such an approach is predicated on the assumption that principals are able to reassure themselves about the agents' ability and willingness to deliver. Competing agents were a key part of the 1990 NHS market reforms (Propper, 1995), with provider units (NHS Trusts – the agents) having to compete for contracts from purchasers (health authorities – the principals).

An elaboration of both these approaches is for principals to build into their relationships with agents incentives (rewards or punishments) for specific behaviours and performance. This can only be done when there are mechanisms available for principals to call agents to account. In general, such calling to account involves measurement and monitoring as a means of diminishing the information asymmetries between principals and agents.

All of these approaches to agent control must of necessity take place against a background of trust. This trust may be in the agents themselves or may be placed in the mechanisms of control. In practice, it is impossible for principals to measure, monitor and verify every aspect of agents' motivations, actions or performance. Even when performance measures are available, or systems of audit are put in place, the principal must, in turn, trust that these provide reliable means of verification. Thus, measurement and checking do not obviate the need for trust but instead demand trust of a different sort (Power, 1997).

The key question then, in the design of performance management and accountability systems, is *what is the appropriate balance between checking and trusting?* A clearer understanding of the nature of checking and trusting may help elucidate this dilemma.

Checking

Measuring and Monitoring Using Performance Indicators

The 1980s and 1990s have seen an inexorable rise in the use of performance indicators in health care (a rise mirrored in the increasing use of indicators in many other parts of the public sector, especially education). By the late 1980s over 2,000 indicators were being produced and circulated to health authorities (Ham and Woolley, 1996). These indicators could be grouped into five main areas: clinical activity, finance, manpower, ambulance services and estate management (ibid.). Composite indicators too (such as the NHS Efficiency Index and the Labour Productivity Index) were also developed to overcome the difficulties of trying to focus on such a large number of individual measures. These composites have been substantially criticized elsewhere (Appleby, 1996a and 1996b) and will not be pursued here. Of greatest interest in this chapter are the indicators of clinical performance.

In the late 1980s and early 1990s there began a gradual disillusionment with measures of clinical activity (process measures) and a growing interest in examining health outcomes. This shift in emphasis came about in part because of renewed political emphasis on 'ends' rather than 'means', and in part because of studies which demonstrated that there was often not much of a link between health care activities and subsequent patient outcomes (Hammermeister et al., 1995; Kazandjian et al., 1995). The new emphasis on outcomes was so powerful, and at times had such an evangelical stridency, that some have dubbed it '*the outcomes movement*' (Delamothe, 1994).

Measuring and monitoring clinical activity (whether process or outcomes) as a precursor to establishing control requires three major stages (Nutley and Smith, 1998). First, data must be collected, second they must be analysed and interpreted and third they must result in action which enhances performance. Problems exist with all three of these stages.

Data Inadequacies

Performance indicators tend to be based around existing data sets. Such routine data systems are however notoriously unreliable. Data collected are frequently shown to be incomplete and inaccurate (Coulter et al., 1989; Johnson et al., 1991; Barrie and Marsh, 1992; Pears et al., 1992). The need to adjust for case-mix and confounding variables (Orchard, 1994) means that many variables are needed for sensible analysis – one analysis used 1,100 patient variables (Shroyer et al., 1995). Yet because routine data systems are relatively inflexible, the available data set may fall a long way short of the ideal. These problems are widespread and enduring (Cleary et al., 1994; Wyatt, 1995).

Interpretation Difficulties

The analysis and interpretation of observational data need considerable care. In order to be useful in assessing performance, it must be possible to make causal inferences from the observed data. In essence, we are looking to attribute poor measured performance to poor actual performance. In practice such causal attribution is often unwarranted (Davies and Crombie, 1999). There are many factors which intervene to weaken the link between actual practice and recorded performance and these problems are especially acute when the indicators measure outcomes (Davies, 1997) (Figure 14.1). Performance indicators which assess the use of evidence-based treatments can offer considerable advantages (Davies and Crombie, 1995; Crombie and Davies, 1998) (Figure 14.2) but even here interpretation problems remain.

Appropriate and Inappropriate Use

A further stumbling block in the effective use of performance measures lies in the confusion over their appropriate use. Too often it is the data collection and analysis stages that consume all the effort and little attention is paid to exactly how the measured indicators will impact on practice (Davies, 1998; Nutley and Smith, 1998). Empirical work shows that in many situations care staff and even managers are unaware of (or are largely disinterested in) the indicators produced (Goddard et al., 1998). Even when attention is paid to published performance data the focus is more usually on identification of

Variations between different health care providers in their reported outcomes may be attributable to a wide range of factors, including:

- *errors in data* – many studies demonstrate that routine data systems are incomplete and inaccurate (Barrie and Marsh, 1992; Wyatt, 1995);
- *source of the data* – data taken from different systems (e.g. administrative versus clinical) may paint a different picture about the outcomes achieved (Hartz and Kuhn, 1994);
- *choice of outcome measured* – services may appear excellent on some measures (e.g. mortality) and poor on others (e.g. morbidity) (Hartz and Kuhn, 1994);
- *characteristics of the measure* – not all health outcomes can be assessed without bias (e.g. physical, psychological and social function), particularly when the findings are attached to performance appraisal;
- *presence of case mix* – different units may see very different patients (Pollack et al., 1991; Iezzoni et al., 1995 and 1996). Differences between units may be attributable to this rather than differences in performance. Adjustment for case-mix will always be incomplete as we can only adjust for *known* prognostic factors;
- *choice of adjustment scheme* – the choice of the adjustment scheme used may influence unit rankings (Iezzoni et al., 1995 and 1996);
- *extent of upstaging* – all adjustment schemes introduce the possibility of upstaging, whereby there is a gradual drift towards labelling patients as being more severe than they might actually be (Murley, 1991; Green and Wintfeld, 1995). The consequence is that risk-adjusted outcomes may (erroneously) appear to improve;
- *chance variability* – chance variability may lead to blameless units being falsely labelled poor (a Type I error), or may provide inappropriate reassurance by mislabelling actually poor performers as merely average (a Type II error).

Figure 14.1 Causal ambiguity between recorded outcomes and actual performance

Source: adapted from Davies and Crombie, 1997.

Process measures examine the utilization of specific health technologies (diagnostic tests, treatments etc.) in specific patient groups. So long as use of these technologies is well-supported by high quality research evidence, such measures offer certain advantages over measurement of health outcomes. In general, process measures are:

- *readily measured* – utilization of health technologies is relatively easily measured without significant bias or error;
- *easily interpreted* – utilization rates of different technologies can readily be interpreted by reference to the evidence base rather than by inter-unit comparisons;
- *sensitive to deficiencies in care* – in comparison to outcome measures, process measures can identify significant deficiencies with much smaller patient numbers (Mant and Hicks, 1995);
- *indicators for action* – failures identified in the process of care provide clear guidance on what must be remedied to improve health care quality.

Figure 14.2 The advantages of using process measures in assessing quality of care

Source: adapted from Crombie and Davies, 1998.

manifestly poor practice rather than on improving practice among the middle rankers. It is unclear at present exactly how information gathered should be built into performance management systems in order to have maximum (beneficial) impact.

Evidence is also accumulating that performance measures can have unanticipated and perhaps unwanted effects: that is, they may distort or even pervert the behaviour of organizations and individuals. Such dysfunctional consequences can range from the mild or even trivial to the serious and lamentable (Figure 14.3). Clearly, given the clandestine nature of these responses, a full and true picture of such practices is unlikely to emerge. Nonetheless, the fact that performance indicators can have deleterious as well as desirable consequences is undeniable and needs to be borne in mind when designing systems to manage performance.

Organizations or individuals may alter their behaviour in response to performance indicators in a variety of undesirable ways:

- *tunnel vision* – concentration on those clinical areas measured to the detriment of other important areas;
- *sub-optimization* – the pursuit of narrow objectives within a unit or organization at the expense of strategic coordination with others;
- *myopia* – concentration on short-term issues and the neglect of long-term criteria;
- *convergence* – an emphasis on not being exposed as an outlier rather than a desire to be outstanding;
- *ossification* – a disinclination to experiment with new and innovative approaches for fear of appearing to perform poorly;
- *gaming* – altering behaviour to gain strategic advantage;
- *misrepresentation* – including creative accounting and fraud.

Figure 14.3 Possible dysfunctional consequences arising from performance indicators

Source: adapted from Smith, 1995a and 1995b.

Finally, even when robust attributions of causality can be made, a fundamental drawback of performance indicators is that they are of necessity backward looking. That is, they report on past performance which (as will be clear from many an advert for financial products) is no guarantee of future performance. Thus using indicators to reward, punish or otherwise compel good practice represents end-of-process error detection rather than pro-active building-in of quality from the beginning.

Checking in Sum

Performance indicators have the potential to reduce some of the reasons for concern over principal-agent relationships. A free flow of information on agent activity and outcomes reduces the asymmetry of information between principal and agent. The provision of such information allows the development of a (perhaps limited) market whereby agents compete to serve principals. Finally, the use of incentives based on performance data can foster a better alignment of goals between principals and their agents. Nonetheless, checking is not the whole story and all principal-agent relationships must to some extent rely on *trust* in order to function.

Trusting

The Necessity of Trust

Full verification of all agent actions and their consequences is simply not possible in any except the most trivial of relationships. It is not the *quantity* of activity that needs checking that poses the problem (sampling would overcome this); it is the variety and *complexity* of the activities of interest which makes checking an incomplete solution. Given the diversity and immeasurability of health care, health service managers and purchasing authorities cannot hope to check everything that matters. For example, formal contracts between principals and agents (e.g. the contracts between health purchasers and NHS trusts) cannot hope to specify in entirety the service desired, and so principals must trust that the aspects unspecified will still be delivered and delivered well. The inevitability of incomplete monitoring means that principals also need to trust that the unmeasured aspects of performance do not become neglected and degraded. Therefore, although trust may not always be openly acknowledged, almost all principal-agent relationships involve at least some trust as a backdrop to more explicit arrangements.

Even in relationships characterized by close scrutiny through detailed performance monitoring, trust is not entirely absent. The principal may be demonstrating a lack of direct trust in the agent (absence of first order trust), but they are nonetheless trusting that the established checking mechanisms (audits or performance measures, for example) are giving a true picture (this is second order trust). Given that trust is ever-present this begs the question of which kind of trust provides the best balance between the costs of checking and the benefits of suppressing opportunistic behaviour?

Types of Trust

Trust as a concept has been of growing interest to social, political and management scientists over recent years. Gambetta's definition provides a useful start in unravelling its nature: trust is the subjective assessment of the probability of action regardless of monitoring (Gambetta, 1988). That is, principals are placing trust in their agent when they come to a judgment that the agent will perform appropriately even when their performance remains unmeasured. Thus trust is a response to the presence of uncertainty and risk which also implies a level of choice: we can choose to trust or we can choose to use other means to encourage action. Trust without an element of choice is merely hope or dependency.

Gambetta's definition highlights the importance of interpersonal relationships in trust. However, trust can also exist between organizations (Lane and Bachmann, 1998). Such trust may or may not be founded on interpersonal relationships – it may, for example, be based on an organization's reputation. Trust can also exist in society as a basic social asset (Fukuyama, 1995). Thus trust acts as a kind of social lubricant, facilitating transactions which would otherwise not be possible or economic. If we can trust, then many of the costly overheads of relationships between principals and agents (transaction costs) are obviated.

Building sufficient trust to allow the reduction of transaction costs may not however be cost-free. It may involve a substantial investment of time and some sunk costs (e.g. building a reputation as a basis for future trust can involve committing resources now for uncertain future benefit). Attempts to build trust may also open up organizations to significant risk of exploitation (i.e. not all attempts to build trust will succeed and those that fail may incur extensive costs).

It is worth noting that there is an asymmetry between trust and distrust. Trust may be difficult and time-consuming to develop, but it is very easily lost and perhaps then even more difficult to regain. A single breach of trust may involve principals moving rapidly to costly checking mechanisms and may leave them reluctant to leave any aspect of agents' performance unspecified or unmeasured. Distrust, should it arise, is also different from a mere absence of trust. Distrust represents an *expectation of exploitative behaviour*, rather than a simple lack of confidence in appropriate action. Thus distrust brings with it a costly necessity of checking in search of reassurance which may be unwarranted. Distrust can, of course, be as misplaced as trust.

Trust in Health Care

There are concerns that social trust is ebbing away in modern developed countries with unclear consequences for social cohesion and institutional performance (Fukuyama, 1995). These concerns are particularly acute in health care. The rise of managed care in the US, with its close control over physician behaviour, has intruded on the previously sacrosanct relationship between patient and doctor. Perhaps as a result, public confidence in doctors has tumbled over recent years (Rodwin, 1993; Mechanic, 1996). In the UK, several high profile cases have contributed to mounting public concern. For example, the 'Child B' case led to much press speculation about the withholding of life-saving treatment (Entwistle et al., 1996), and the recent General Medical Council disciplinary hearing into three Bristol doctors highlighted poor outcomes after paediatric cardiac surgery (Smith, 1998). Such cases have undoubtedly led to a diminution of public trust in both doctors and the NHS (Davies and Shields, 1999).

Despite concerns over falling levels of social trust, at least some of new Labour's policies in the NHS are predicated on the existence of trust between different parts of the health service. For example, the move away from (quasi-) competition and towards cooperation and contestability (Ham, 1996) in the contractual relationship between health authorities and NHS trusts signifies a tacit acceptance that trust matters (Goddard and Mannion, 1998). In addition, empirical work in the wake of the UK government's 'Community Care' reforms showed that – in the absence of firm data – reputation and trust were central to the operation of the community care market (Mannion and Smith, 1997).

Trust figures in many other relationships within health care. For example, professional self-regulation within medicine (now under considerable strain (Klein, 1998)) embodies trust (or perhaps something closer to dependency). However, the role of trust in the smooth functioning of health systems has yet to be fully articulated or systematically explored empirically.

Trust and Performance

The utilization of trust has come to be seen by some as an invigorating concept for business (Whitney, 1993; Lane and Bachmann, 1998). The best modern business organizations are flatter, less hierarchical and less reliant on measurement. They emphasize empowerment of human individuals, and try to implement the features of 'learning organizations' (Garvin, 1993; Sewell, 1997).

There is some evidence that actions which imply a lack of trust (such as performance-related pay) may actually diminish performance by displacing intrinsic motivations (Osterloh and Frey, 1998). However, contexts when this will occur are largely undetermined. Use of performance indicators, especially when published, can certainly imply a lack of trust in professionalism (Davies and Lampel, 1998) and may thus impact deleteriously on performance. This issue needs additional study. Further, it is not yet apparent whether trust exists within organizations which are high performers *because* they are high performers, or whether trust can of itself *lead* to improved performance. That is, the direction of causality for any associations found between trust and performance is unsettled. Thus, the crucial relationship between trust and performance remains unclear and in urgent need of clarification.

Trust in Sum

Despite the upsurge of interest in trust over recent years, and a more explicit recognition of its role within and between well-functioning organization, much remains unclear. Trust may be efficient in many circumstances because of reduced transaction costs compared to checking. In other circumstances it would be foolhardy: the world is not populated exclusively with saints (Kay, 1992). So the down side of trust is the potential for unchecked inadequate performance or naked opportunism.

That trust is an unavoidable part of the fabric of principal-agent relationships is apparent. It also closely bound up with those intangible aspects of agents such as reputation. But what this means for effective systems of performance management and clinical accountability is not yet clear. Nonetheless, issues of trust cannot be ignored just because they are difficult. A headlong rush for the obvious benefits of checking may be misplaced (Davies and Lampel, 1998).

Concluding Remarks

Recent high profile failures of both performance and accountability (most notably, the disastrous mortality rates of two Bristol-base paediatric cardiac surgeons (Smith, 1998) and failures in cervical cancer screening services (Miller, 1995)) have served only to emphasize the need for effective mechanisms to ensure quality. In any such discussions over performance management the need for performance measurement (and appropriate incentive contexts) usually figures large. However, there exist different ways in which the principal-agent problem can be overcome, each with a distinctive set of advantages, costs and drawbacks. Over-reliance on any one approach is likely to make its deficiencies more apparent (Hood, 1995). Therefore the key issue remains of how to balance the different approaches to best effect.

Checking, in the form of measurement and monitoring linked to punishment and rewards, has palpable appeal. Trusting seems less intuitive, more hazardous, fragile and even embarrassingly naive. However, unless we understand its important role in maintaining and improving performance we may fail to appreciate its value until after its demise. As clinical governance is clarified in the UK, and managed care organizations in the US seek more varied methods of control, a number of considerations need to be kept to the fore.

One Size Does Not Fit All

One obvious fact to emerge from the preceding discussion is that any approach to performance management may work *for some services, some of the time.* No single approach is likely to be a panacea. For example, what works for surgical specialities may be inappropriate for mental health services; different systems might be needed to ensure basic competence, compared to those needed to foster clinical excellence; and different approaches may be tried during periods of stability compared to times of rapid structural change. Unravelling the contexts within which different approaches are either effectual or counterproductive will allow more sophisticated and selective performance management.

Instrumentality is Not Assured

The linkage between data and actions is often largely ignored in the design of performance systems (Nutley and Smith, 1998; Davies, 1998). Because of this the impact of such systems may be minimal. The people whose practice is under scrutiny, and those whose actions can influence change, need to be identified and drawn into the systems, preferably at the design stage. Without interest and ownership of performance systems by those who the system is intended to influence, such systems may be seen as irrelevant or may be used simply to identify manifest failures (Goddard et al., 1998).

Incentives May have Unintended Effects

The incentive context surrounding any measurement will sometimes influence behaviour and sometimes not. More unfortunately, it will sometimes influence behaviour in undesirable directions. Thus, in developing any systems of measurement as a precursor to control, careful consideration of the full incentive context is needed to identify likely impacts and reverse effects. The incentive context is much wider than financial rewards or punishments. For example, it also encompasses impacts on status, reputation and work satisfaction. Clarifying the incentive context and ensuring that there are no unanticipated spill-over effects (perhaps arising from publication of performance information) is not straightforward.

Measurement Offers Only a Partial Picture

Hard data paint only a part of the picture on performance. Soft qualitative information on such issues as reputation are also a very important part of the way in which people make judgments (Mannion and Smith, 1997). We have yet to understand how best to capitalize on such information in making judgments and identifying areas for quality improvement. Such lack of understanding should not, however, blind us to the important role played by non-measured factors.

Trust is a Must

Finally, health care professionals have much tacit knowledge and expertise not readily condensed and codified. Therefore any measurement system is of necessity incomplete, leaving always a large margin for trust. Recognizing this and its importance may allow a richer understanding of how best to manage clinical performance and assure professional accountability. The challenge is to know when and how to trust, and when and how to check.[1]

Note

1   The authors would like to thank many people for insightful discussions of these issues over many years. They are particularly grateful to: Maria Goddard, Joseph Lampel, Sandra Nutley, Pete Smith, Manouche Tavakoli, Richard Thomson and Kieran Walshe. Naturally, the authors alone take full responsibility for the content.

One author (Huw Davies) held the position as *Harkness Fellow in Health Care Policy* during the preparation of this chapter. Thus this work was supported by The Commonwealth Fund, a New York city-based private independent foundation. However, the views presented here are those of the authors and not necessarily those of The Commonwealth Fund, its directors, officers or staff. Huw Davies is immensely grateful to The Fund for the opportunities afforded him by the Fellowship.

References

Appleby, J. (1996a), *A Measure of Effectiveness? A critical review of the NHS Efficiency Index*, NAHAT, Birmingham.

Appleby, J. (1996b), 'Promoting Efficiency in the NHS: Problems with the labour productivity index', *British Medical Journal*, 313, pp. 1319–21.

Barrie, J.L. and Marsh, D.R. (1992), 'Quality of Data in the Manchester Orthopaedic Database', *British Medical Journal*, 304, pp. 159–62.

Cleary, R., Beard, R., Coles, J., Devlin, B., Hopkins, A., Schumacher, D. and Wickings, I. (1994), 'Comparative Hospital Databases: Value for management and quality', *Quality in Health Care*, 3, pp. 3–10.

Coulter, A., Brown, S. and Daniels, A. (1989), 'Computer Held Chronic Disease Registers in General Practice: A validation study', *Journal of Epidemiology and Community Health*, 43, pp. 25–8.

Crombie, I.K. and Davies, H.T.O. (1998), 'Beyond Health Outcomes: The advantages of measuring process', *Journal of Evaluation in Clinical Practice*, 4, pp. 31–8.

Davies, H.T.O. (1997), 'What's a Healthy Outcome?', *Health Service Journal*, 107 (5548), p. 22.

Davies, H.T.O. (1998), 'Performance Management Using Health Outcomes: In search of instrumentality', *Journal of Evaluation in Clinical Practice*, 4, pp. 150–3.

Davies, H.T.O. and Crombie, I.K. (1995), 'Assessing the Quality of Care: Measuring well supported processes may be more enlightening than monitoring outcomes', *British Medical Journal*, 311, p. 766.

Davies, H.T.O. and Crombie, I.K. (1997), 'Interpreting Health Outcomes', *Journal of Evaluation in Clinical Practice*, 3, pp. 187–200.

Davies, H.T.O. and Crombie, I.K. (1999), 'Outcomes from Observational Studies: Understanding causal ambiguity', *Drug Information Journal* (in press).

Davies, H.T.O. and Lampel, J. (1998), 'Trust in Performance Indicators', *Quality in Health Care*, 7, pp. 159–62.

Davies, H.T.O. and Shields, A. (1999), 'Public Trust, and Accountability for Clinical Performance: Lessons from the media reporting of the Bristol enquiry' (in manuscript form, available from the author).

Delamothe, T. (1994), 'Preface' in T. Delamothe (ed.), *Outcomes into Clinical Practice*, BMJ Publishing Group, London.

Entwistle, V.A., Watt, I.S., Bradbury, R. and Pehl, L.J. (1996), 'Media Coverage of the Child B Case', *British Medical Journal*, 312, pp. 1587–91.

Fukuyama, F. (1995), *Trust: The social virtues and the creation of prosperity*, The Free Press, New York.

Gambetta, D. (1988), *Trust: Making and breaking co-operative relations*, Blackwell, Oxford.

Garvin, D.A. (1993), 'Building a Learning Organization', *Harvard Business Review*, 71, pp. 78–91.

Goddard, M. and Mannion, M. (1998), 'From Competition to Co-operation: New economic relationships in the National Health Service', *Health Economics*, 7, pp. 105–19.

Goddard, M., Mannion, R. and Smith, P.C. (1998), 'All Quiet on the Front Line', *Health Service Journal*, pp. 24–6.

Green, J. and Wintfeld, N. (1995), 'Report Cards on Cardiac Surgeons: Assessing New York State's Approach', *New England Journal of Medicine*, 332, pp. 1229–32.

Ham, C. (1996), 'Contestability: A middle path for health care', *British Medical Journal*, 312, pp. 70–1.

Ham, C. and Woolley, M. (1996), *How Does the NHS measure up? Assessing the performance of health authorities*, NAHAT, Birmingham.

Hammermeister, K.E., Shroyer, A.L., Sethi, G.K. and Grover, F.L. (1995), 'Why it is Important to Demonstrate Linkages Between Outcomes of Care and Processes and Structures of Care', *Medical Care*, 33, pp. OS5–16.

Hartz, A.J. and Kuhn, E.M. (1994), 'Comparing Hospitals That Perform Coronary Artery Bypass Surgery: The Effect of Outcome Measures and Data Sources', *American Journal of Public Health*, 84, pp. 1609–14.

Hood, C. (1995), 'Controlling Public Management', *Public Finance Foundation Review*, 7, pp. 3–6.

Iezzoni, L.I., Shwartz, M., Ash, A.S., Hughes, J.S., Daley, J. and Mackiernan, Y.D. (1995), 'Using Severity-adjusted Stroke Mortality Rates to Judge Hospitals', *International Journal for Quality in Health Care*, 7, pp. 81–94.

Iezzoni, L.I., Shwartz, M., Ash, A.S., Hughes, J.S., Daley, J. and Mackiernan, Y.D. (1996), 'Severity Measurement Methods and Judging Hospital Death Rates for Pneumonia', *Medical Care*, 34, pp. 11–28.

Johnson, N., Mant, D., Jones, L. and Randall, T. (1991), 'Use of Computerised General Practice Data for Population Surveillance: Comparative study of influenza data', *British Medical Journal*, 302, pp. 763–5.

Kay, N.M. (1992), 'Markets, False Hierarchies and the Evolution of the Modern Corporation', *Journal of Economic Behavior and Organization*, 17, pp. 315–33.

Kazandjian, V.A., Wood, P. and Lawthers, J. (1995), 'Balancing Science and Practice in Indicator Development: The Maryland Hospital Association Quality Indicator (QI) Project', *International Journal for Quality in Health Care*, 7, pp. 39–46.

Klein, R. (1998), 'Competence, Professional Self Regulation, and the Public Interest', *British Medical Journal*, 316, pp. 1740–2.

Lane, C. and Bachmann, R. (ed.) (1998), *Trust Within and Between Organizations*, Oxford University Press, Oxford.

Mannion, R. and Smith, P.C. (1997), 'Trust and Reputation in Community Care: Theory and evidence' in P. Anand and A. McGuire (eds), *Changes in Health Care: Reflections on the NHS internal market*, Macmillan Business, Basingstoke.

Mant, J. and Hicks, N. (1995), 'Detecting Differences in Quality of Care: How sensitive are process and outcome measures in the treatment of acute myocardial infarction?', *British Medical Journal*, 311, pp. 793–6.

Mechanic, D. (1996), 'Changing Medical Organization and the Erosion of Trust', *Milbank Quarterly*, 74, pp. 171–89.

Miller, A.B. (1995), 'Failures of Cervical Cancer Screening', editorial, *American Journal of Public Health*, 85, pp. 761–2.

Murley, R.S. (1991), 'Axillary Dissection in Breast Cancer', *Lancet*, 337, pp. 1221.

NHS Executive (1998),*The New NHS: Modern and Dependable. A National Framework for Assessing Performance*, Leeds, NHS Executive.

Nutley, S. and Smith, P. (1998), 'League Tables for Performance Improvement in Health Care', *Journal of Health Services Research and Policy*, 3, pp. 50–7.

Orchard, C. (1994), 'Comparing Healthcare Outcomes', *British Medical Journal*, 308, pp. 1493–6.

Osterloh, M. and Frey, B.S. (1998), 'Does Pay for Performance Really Motivate Employees?' in A.D. Neely and D.B. Waggoner (eds), *Performance Measurement – Theory and Practice*, Cambridge University Press, Cambridge.

Pears, J., Alexander, V., Alexander, G.F. and Waugh, N.R. (1992), 'Audit of the Quality of Hospital Discharge Data', *Health Bulletin (Edinburgh)*, 50, pp. 356–61.

Pollack, M.M., Alexander, S.R., Clarke, N., Ruttimann, U.E., Tesselaar, H.M. and Bachulis, A.C. (1991), 'Improved Outcomes from Tertiary Center Pediatric Intensive Care: A statewide comparison of tertiary and nontertiary care facilities', *Critical Care Medicine*, 19, pp. 150–9.

Power, M. (1997), *The Audit Society: Rituals of Verification*, Oxford University Press, Oxford.

Propper, C. (1995), 'Agency and Incentives in the NHS Internal Narket', *Soc Sci Med*, 40, pp. 1683–90.

Robinson, R. and Steiner, A. (1998), *Managed Health Care*, Open University Press, Buckingham.

Rodwin, M. (1993), *Medicine, Money and Morals: Physicians' conflicts of interest*, Oxford University Press, New York.

Secretary of State for Health (1998),*A First Class Service: Quality in the new NHS*, Department of Health, London.

Secretary of State for Health (1998), *The New NHS: Modern and Dependable*, HMSO, London.

Sewell, N. (1997), 'Do You Work in a Learning or Improving Organisation?', *British Journal of Health Care Management*, 3, pp. 315–7.

Shroyer, A.L., London, M.J., Sethi, G.K., Marshall, G., Grover, F.L. and Hammermeister, K.E. (1995), 'Relationships between Patient-related Risk Factors, Processes, Structures, and Outcomes of Cardiac Surgical Care. Conceptual Models', *Medical Care*, 33, pp. OS26–34.

Smith, P. (1995), 'On the Unintended Consequences of Publishing Performance Data in the Public Sector', *International Journal of Public Administration*, 18, pp. 277–310.

Smith, P. (1995), 'Outcome-related Performance Indicators and Organizational Control in the Public Sector' in J. Holloway, J. Lewis and G. Mallory (eds), *Performance Measurement and Evaluation*, SAGE, London.

Smith, P.C., Stepan, A., Valdmanis, V. and Verheyen, P. (1997), 'Principal-agent Problems in Health Care Systems: An international perspective', *Health Policy*, 41, pp. 37–60.

Smith, R. (1998), 'All Changed, Changed Utterly', *British Medical Journal*, 316, pp. 1917–8.

Whitney, J.O. (1993), *The Economics of Trust: Liberating profits and restoring corporate vitality*, McGraw-Hill, New York.

Wyatt, J. (1995), 'Acquisition and Use of Clinical Data for Audit and Research', *Journal of Evaluation in Clinical Practice*, 1, pp. 15–27.

List of Contributors

Elizabeth M. Alder

Department of Epidemiology and Public Health, Ninewells Medical School, Dundee

Juan I. Baeza

Centre for Health Services Studies, University of Kent

Régis Blais

Groupe de recherche interdisciplinaire en santé, Faculté de médecine, Université de Montréal and Département d'administration de la santé, Faculté de médecine, Université de Montréal

Pierre Boyle

Département de médecine sociale et préventive, Faculté de médecine, Université de Montréal

Michael Calnan

Centre for Health Services Studies, University of Kent

David Cline

CRAG Secretariat, Edinburgh

Iain K. Crombie

Department of Epidemiology and Public Health, University of Dundee, Ninewells Hospital and Medical School, Dundee

Huw T.O. Davies

Department of Management, University of St Andrews

John L. Deffenbaugh

Frontline Management Consultants, Stirling

Managing Quality: Strategic Issues in Health Care Management, H.T.O. Davies, M. Tavakoli, M. Malek, A.R. Neilson (eds), Ashgate Publishing Ltd, 1999.

231

Serge Dubé   *Département de chirurgie, Hôpital*
                            Maisonneuve-Rosemont

Dafydd Evans   *Dundee Dental School*

Alan Finlayson   *ISD Scotland, Edinburgh*

Moira Fischbacher   *Department of Management Studies,*
                            University of Glasgow Business School

Arthur Francis   *University of Bradford Management Centre*

Colin Gordon   *Health Economics Research Unit,*
                            University of Aberdeen

Mike Hart   *King Alfred's University College,*
                            Winchester

Gail Johnston   *Department of General Practice, Queen's*
                            University of Belfast

Steve Kendrick   *ISD Scotland, Edinburgh*

Joanne Lally   *Department of Epidemiology and Public*
                            Health, School of Health Sciences, The
                            Medical School, University of Newcastle

Danielle Larouche   *Groupe de recherche interdisciplinaire en*
                            santé, Faculté de médecine, Université de
                            Montréal

Anne Ludbrook   *Health Economics Research Unit,*
                            University of Aberdeen

Mo Malek   *Department of Management, University of*
                            St Andrews

Russell Mannion   *Centre for Health Economics, University of*
                            York

Andrew R. Millard   *Scottish Clinical Audit Resource Centre, University of Glasgow*

Aileen Neilson   *Department of Management, University of St Andrews*

Sandra Nutley   *Department of Management, University of St Andrews*

Raynald Pineault   *Groupe de recherche interdisciplinaire en santé, Faculté de médecine, Université de Montréal and Département de médecine sociale et préventive, Faculté de médecine, Université de Montréal*

Chris Southwick   *General Dental Practitioner, Dundee*

Manouche Tavakoli   *Department of Management, St Andrews University*

Richard Thomson   *UK QIP*

Mike Walsh   *Faculty of Health, University of Hull*

Richard Wilson   *Department of Public Health and Epidemiology, Medical School, University of Birmingham*